Mental Health and Poverty

Mental Health and Poverty

Rob Poole

Professor of Social Psychiatry, School of Social Sciences, Bangor University;
Co-Director, Centre for Mental Health and Society, Wales; and Honorary
Consultant Psychiatrist, Betsi Cadwaladr University Health Board

Robert Higgo

Consultant Psychiatrist, Mersey Care NHS Trust, Liverpool; Honorary
Research Fellow, School of Social Sciences, Bangor University; and
Associate Member, Centre for Mental Health and Society, Wales

Catherine A. Robinson

Professor of Social Policy Research, School of Social Sciences, Bangor
University; and Co-Director, Centre for Mental Health and Society,
Wales

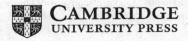
CAMBRIDGE
UNIVERSITY PRESS

CAMBRIDGE
UNIVERSITY PRESS

University Printing House, Cambridge CB2 8BS, United Kingdom

Published in the United States of America by Cambridge University Press, New York

Cambridge University Press is part of the University of Cambridge.

It furthers the University's mission by disseminating knowledge in the pursuit of education, learning and research at the highest international levels of excellence.

www.cambridge.org
Information on this title: www.cambridge.org/9780521143967

First published 2014

A catalogue record for this publication is available from the British Library

Library of Congress Cataloguing in Publication data
Poole, Rob, 1956–
Mental health and poverty / Rob Poole, Robert Higgo, Catherine A. Robinson.
   pages   cm
Includes bibliographical references and index.
ISBN 978-0-521-14396-7 (hardback)
1. Poor – Mental health.   2. Poverty – Health aspects.   3. Mental health – Social aspects.
4. Mental illness – Economic aspects.   I. Higgo, Robert, 1952–   II. Title.
RC451.4.P6P66   2014
616.890086'942 – dc23 .   2013032647

ISBN 978-0-521-14396-7 Hardback

....

This book is dedicated to the late Aneurin Bevan, founder of the National Health Service, who once said 'If freedom is to be saved and enlarged, poverty must be ended. There is no other solution' (Bevan, 1952).

Contents

Acknowledgements

RP and RH started writing this book four years ago, with the firm intention that it would be completed within two years. It proved more difficult to write than we expected, and there were times when it seemed unlikely that we would ever finish it at all. In the final year, CAR joined us and we started again from scratch. The process started with a marathon and ended with a sprint. We have tested the patience of Richard Marley of Cambridge University Press, who nonetheless has remained unfailingly supportive. We value his loyalty and we are seriously considering paying for his dinner next time we meet.

Many of the ideas set out in this book were developed in the course of long discussions and debates with our university and NHS colleagues. We acknowledge their role in sharpening our thinking. We are particularly grateful to Gordon Kennedy, Dr Theresa McArdle and Dr Sue Ruben, who read an earlier draft and passed helpful comments. Sue Ruben also assisted by loaning us her cottage, which was fittingly named Pentop. She painted the cover illustration. Steve Hammond of Hammond Design Ltd turned this into a high quality digital image. The text benefited from skilful copy-editing by Zoë Lewin who was consistently patient and helpful.

Latterly we wrote as a threesome at a variety of locations in mid-Wales. This entailed complex and ever changing arrangements, which were uncomplainingly organised by Sue Jones. We thank her for her skill in herding cats.

Finally, we have greatly benefitted from the support and forbearance of our families, some of whom have had to cook for themselves in our absence.

Preface

Serious mental illness is a disease of poverty in much the same way as cholera or tuberculosis. Anyone can suffer from these illnesses, but people are much more likely to do so if they are poor.

People living in poverty tend to experience worse outcomes from treatment than wealthier people.

A substantial part of clinical practice for most mental health professionals involves effort to help patients to overcome the extensive adverse effects of social deprivation.

The most important measure that might plausibly reduce the incidence and prevalence of serious mental illness is action to reduce poverty and income inequality.

Intervention at an individual level is unlikely to prevent mental illness, but action against poverty would be a powerful public health measure.

The purpose of this book is to explore the evidence that tends to support these statements, paying due attention to the ambiguities in the literature. We examine the scientific, policy and clinical implications of the knowledge base on poverty for practising mental health professionals.

Two of us have previously written two books about clinical skills (Poole & Higgo, 2006, 2008). This book is a dissimilar exercise with a different authorship. Catherine Robinson has brought a social science perspective, together with new ways of thinking about the material. She has driven us to a systematic, closely referenced approach that is more scholarly than our previous texts.

When this book was first being developed it seemed to be an idea that already existed independently of us, a glaring gap in the market. There was, we thought, an obvious need for a readable but scientifically sound book that drew out the strength of the evidence about the social origins of major mental illness. It seemed particularly appropriate to write the book at a time when widespread disillusionment had set in over the very limited results of the alleged biological revolution of the 1990s. It had been promised that new genetics and new pharmacology would transform clinical practice in psychiatry. Instead, service delivery systems have been transformed, but the actual treatments given to patients looked remarkably similar to those being offered 20 years earlier. A new wave of enthusiasm for social psychiatry was developing. The time was right, the theme was right and we had the necessary skills within the new authorship.

The task was, however, daunting. There was a huge amount of material to review, but we retained a commitment to write books that would be read rather than consulted. We have produced a book that is relatively short. We have not systematically reviewed the whole of the massive literature that is relevant to our main themes. Had we done so, each of the chapters herein would have been several hundred pages long. Even if we had the resources to produce such a tome, a densely and meticulously referenced text would be unlikely to achieve our primary objective, which is to draw attention to an aspect of psychiatry that is entirely obvious in clinical practice, but until relatively recently has been neglected within psychiatric journals and textbooks.

There is a marked skew in this book towards discussion of the socio-economic factors associated with schizophrenia rather than other mental disorders. We do not apologise for this, as schizophrenia is the diagnosis where the evidence is strongest and most extensive. However, we must warn readers that we move between discussion of different diagnostic categories. Terms such as schizophrenia, psychosis, and psychotic symptoms are not synonyms. Each has been used to convey a different meaning, which we hope is evident from careful attention to the text.

Although there is an unmistakable rhetorical flow to this book, we maintain a strong attachment to evidence and empiricism. We have endeavoured to achieve a balanced overview, without exaggerating the strength of our argument. We explore some parts of the evidence in detail. We have not attempted to smooth over a number of contradictions. We have tried to draw a clear distinction between our opinions and sustainable facts.

This text follows the model of the previous Poole & Higgo books in that it is strongly influenced by the experience of two social psychiatrists with many long years of inner-city practice behind them. Catherine Robinson is a social scientist with a strong background in service user and carer research. The three of us share an interest in narrative as a tool of empiricism. However, we offer no novel insights or conceptual innovations here. The UK produces much of the best social psychiatry research in the world, and we embrace that tradition. Our collective research interests are somewhat closer to social science than biomedical methods.

Alongside our wish to draw attention to what is already known about the relationship between mental illness and poverty, we have a secondary objective, which is to draw out and articulate the nature and principles of modern social psychiatry in clinical practice. We feel that in recent years this important theoretical orientation has tended to lack the strident advocacy evident in the biological and psychological traditions, despite a high level of research activity.

We have been surprised and pleased that the previous Poole & Higgo books have been well received, not just by psychiatrists, but also by nurses and social workers. This has occurred despite our defence of a version of the medical model. We hope that this will prove to be the case again. Some readers with a background in public health or sociology will probably be dismayed to find that a book with the term 'mental health' in the title is almost entirely devoted to issues concerning serious mental illness. There is only limited discussion of the positive health and well-being agenda. What we have to say on that subject is likely to prove controversial. Nonetheless it has seemed to us to be appropriate to retain 'mental health' in the title. We have serious misgivings over conflating mental health with well-being, and even greater misgivings over attempts by mental health professionals to promote happiness rather than to relieve suffering. We believe that there is good reason to suppose that a significant proportion of people who are vulnerable to serious mental illness would remain in good mental health if measures were taken to tackle poverty and inequality.

Just as the contract for this book was being agreed with Cambridge University Press, Wilkinson and Pickett's *The Spirit Level* (Wilkinson & Pickett, 2009) was published. This has had a major impact in bringing the issue of income inequality to the centre of debate about health inequalities. We acknowledge the importance of Wilkinson and Pickett's work to our own thinking. It is fortuitous that their book has had the effect of making ours more topical.

Little in this book will seem particularly radical to social scientists. Within psychiatry, however, the suggestion that the most important measure that would improve public mental health would be steps to reduce inequality sounds suspiciously political. None of us belongs to a political party. It would be disingenuous to deny that we have a strong attachment to social justice and that we have little sympathy with the neo-liberal economic orthodoxies of our time. However, this book is not driven by the demands of ideology. It is driven by evidence and by experience. Our attachment to scientific empiricism is stronger than our attachment to any set of political ideas. As a consequence we recognise that many of our most cherished ideas about mental illness will, in the fullness of time, be shown to be simplistic or plain wrong, including some of those set out here. We are not 'radical psychiatrists' or 'radical social scientists'. If the evidence leads us to conclusions that seem radical, this reflects the strange position that UK political thought has arrived at in the twenty-first century, with a set of values that are based upon a seemingly unchallengeable assertion that there is no alternative to unbridled market capitalism. It is hard to believe that over the past 30 years it has been part of the orthodoxy of mainstream UK political parties that worsening social inequality is either inevitable or actually a good thing.

In denying radical intent, there is a danger that we might be thought to have produced a work that is fundamentally inconsequential. The existence of a connection between poverty and emotional distress appears to be quite obvious, and in no way surprising. Common sense would dictate that it is self-evident that children who grow up in the poorest neighbourhoods, and in the poorest families within those areas, are much more likely to become unhappy adults than children who grow up in privilege. There are many aphorisms to the effect that money doesn't make you happy, but experience suggests otherwise. Readers are invited to compare and contrast The Beatles' *Can't Buy Me Love* with Randy Newman's *It's Money That I Love*. The arguments in the latter appear to us to be more robust.

Common sense is not always reliable. The relationship between adversity and mental ill health is much more complex than simple truisms might suggest. Many of the well established associations between poverty and mental ill health are strongly counter-intuitive. For example, whilst Marx (Marx & Engels, 2008) believed that capitalism had rescued the nineteenth century working class from the '*idiocy of rural existence*', it appears to be less harmful to grow up in rural poverty than urban poverty.

We are discomfited that some of the content of this book could be taken to portray people in lower socio-economic classes as passive victims, in need of rescue by paternalistic philanthropy. This is not in accordance with our experience of working in a deprived inner city, where people's resourcefulness, sense of community and optimism is often inspiring. Our recognition of the socio-economic factors that cause and shape mental disorder does not contradict the abiding principle that mental health professionals are most helpful to patients when they get alongside them and their communities.

Rob Poole
Robert Higgo
Catherine A. Robinson
May 2013

Severe mental illness and social factors

This chapter examines the evidence about the relationship between poverty and severe mental illness, by which we mean psychotic disorders. In Chapters 2 and 3 the nature of poverty in the UK in the twenty-first century is discussed in detail. It is important to recognise from the outset that the concept of poverty is complex. Individual income is difficult to measure, and may not be as relevant as relative income, perceived disadvantage or social exclusion. It is easy to inadvertently conflate these concepts, and this is apparent in parts of the literature. In this chapter, some work is cited that uses the concepts of social disadvantage and deprivation rather than poverty per se. The movement between discussion of different types of social adversity should not be taken to imply that the differences between them are irrelevant.

On the face of it, it appears self-evident that being poor is bad for people's health. A strong association between poverty and ill health is well established for nearly all types of disease and in all parts of the world (Black *et al.*, 1993). The association between material deprivation and mental illness is just as strong as it is for physical illness. However, it is by no means universally accepted that this relationship is causal; that exposure to poverty leads to mental ill health. Much of the discussion in the psychiatric literature has taken social factors to have a modulating effect on more profoundly causative bio-genetic factors. It is only recently that the possibility of a strictly causal role for social factors has been seriously addressed within the mainstream psychiatric research literature. There is a body of opinion that has long preferred the view that a reverse causation applies, that mental illness causes poverty. The suggestion is that mental illness undermines people's ability to work and to maintain their social position.

Interest in non-biological factors has sharply increased in recent years with regard to schizophrenia in particular. The association between this disorder and social factors is very strong and consistent. A particular type of social factor, namely growing up in inner-city deprivation, seems to be especially powerful in conferring a heightened risk of schizophreniform disorders. For this reason we shall concentrate here on the evidence regarding schizophrenia.

Mental illness and social environment

The theoretical orientation of British psychiatric practice and research has tended to be stable over long periods of time compared with the radical shifts in stance seen in US psychiatry. In Britain there has been a strong biomedical emphasis, with an accompanying interest in social environment that may reflect a pragmatism in our national intellectual traditions. The contemporary American emphasis on the biological, memorably described by a president of the American Psychiatric Association as the *bio-bio-bio* model (Sharfstein, 2005), appears strident and unbalanced from our perspective. It is easy to forget that not so long ago US psychiatry was dominated by psychoanalytic ideas, and that prior to that the US pioneered social psychiatry. In the twentieth century, social psychiatry entered the UK through the influence of an American, Adolph Meyer, on an Australian, Sir Aubrey Lewis (Shepherd, 1996). The UK may lead social psychiatry research now, but the tradition was born in the USA.

The systematic study of the social epidemiology of mental illness starts in the 1930s with the seminal work by Faris and Dunham in Chicago (Faris & Dunham, 1939). Using routinely collected information, they found that schizophrenia was far more common in the 'disorganised areas near the centre of the city' than in the suburbs (respective prevalences of 362/100,000 versus 55.4/100,000). They found a similar but less marked difference in the prevalence of 'senile psychoses and psychosis with arteriosclerosis' (in other words, dementia). They found no such difference in the prevalence of 'manic-depressive insanity'. They were interested in social causation. They reported that catatonic presentations of schizophrenia were commoner in the 'foreign born and Negro slum areas where poverty and culture conflict are combined', whilst paranoid and hebephrenic presentations were commoner 'in the rooming house areas of the city where the primary group has broken down and individuals live in social isolation'. At the time there was much debate about the meaning of these findings, but the idea that gained greatest currency was that living in social isolation in an inner city had a special role in provoking schizophrenia.

In 1956, Edward Hare published a study of the distribution of people diagnosed as suffering from mental illness in Bristol (Hare, 1956). Nearly 60 years after its publication this stands out as a high quality piece of social psychiatry research that identifies many of the methodological problems and core theoretical issues inherent to this field of research. Hare essentially attempted to replicate the work of Faris and Dunham. He recognised that there were some advantages in studying the epidemiology of mental illness in the UK. At that time the degree of social inequality in the UK was less extreme than in the USA, and the existence of a National Health Service that was used by a large proportion of the whole population meant that routinely collected information was likely to be more inclusive.

Hare gained access to the records of the public and private psychiatric hospitals serving the city of Bristol. He collected information on everyone who was admitted for the first time between 1949 and 1953. The period straddled 1951, which was a year when a national census was conducted. The returns from this census gave socio-economic information by electoral ward (the smallest geographical administrative unit in the UK). Hare took the clinical diagnoses given to the patients and put them into five categories: schizophrenia, manic-depressive psychosis (which included severe depression), neurosis, senile dementia, and other (including alcoholism, personality disorder and epileptic disorders). He correlated the prevalence of these diagnoses with three social factors by electoral ward and for three large 'natural communities' within Bristol. The factors were:

- The proportion of single person households in the area. This was taken to be a rough measure of social isolation.
- Mean rateable (property tax) value of property in the area. This was based on an estimate of the notional value of the property, and could be taken to measure the social desirability and the wealth of the area.
- Population density. At the time this could not be easily derived from census data, and Hare had to use a sophisticated method to allow for, for example, the presence of parks in areas of otherwise high population density.

Hare acknowledged the limitations inherent to his research method, and these have continued to be apparent in later research using similar approaches. He had to rely on routinely collected data. When this was analysed and made available by the Office for National Statistics, it was organised by electoral ward. Electoral wards are not natural communities, and often have marked social heterogeneity within them. This can obscure important differences within the ward or across wards. He had to accept clinical diagnoses that may not have been made in a consistent way; this was 1956, many years before the development of structured clinical interviews or diagnostic criteria. As the data depended on contact with services, it is possible that there were differences in the proportions of people with mental illness who presented for treatment in different areas, which would create an apparent difference in prevalence.

In keeping with every other rigorous study conducted in the developed world that has ever been published, Hare found a markedly higher rate of schizophrenia in the inner-city area than elsewhere. He found no differences between areas in the rates of manic-depression, dementia or neurosis. He found that there was a strong association between rates of schizophrenia and living alone. This held true in areas of low and high rateable value and high and low population density.

There is much in Hare's study that is of historical interest. For example, he found the lowest rate of schizophrenia in suburban council estates. This would be unlikely to be true today, as the social composition and structure of social housing estates has changed markedly. His central conclusion was that two factors might account for his findings. Firstly, there might be a causal factor related to social isolation. Secondly, people with schizophrenia might be drawn to live in single person accommodation, which is concentrated in the inner city. Hare did not regard these possibilities as mutually exclusive.

The subsequent literature has not confirmed Hare's findings in their entirety, but debate has continued over his two explanatory possibilities: people with latent or florid schizophrenia drift into poor social conditions (social drift) or certain types of social environment create a vulnerability to, or cause, schizophrenia. Attention has tended to focus on schizophrenia, because the social effect has appeared greatest for this condition. Whilst there is evidence that social deprivation is associated with mental illness of nearly all types, findings are less consistent for other disorders.

Social drift and urban drift

For a long time most psychiatrists believed that the question of social causation of schizophrenia was settled. In part this was because a paper published in 1963 seemed to have convincingly demonstrated that the association between deprivation and schizophrenia was due to social drift (Goldberg & Morrison, 1963). This described an impressively rigorous study with two arms. At that time the General Register Office was routinely notified of the name, date of birth, occupation and diagnosis of every patient admitted to a mental hospital in England and Wales. From these records a sample was taken of men aged between 20 and 34 years who were admitted to hospital for the first time in 1956 with a diagnosis of schizophrenia. Their centrally held birth certificates were examined. These included a record of the father's occupation at the time of the patient's birth. Thus it was possible to compare patients' socio-economic class (SEC) at the time of admission with their fathers' SEC at the time of their birth. The distribution of the fathers' SEC closely matched that of the UK population as a whole. The distribution of the patients' SEC showed a strong skew towards SEC V (manual and unskilled). This appeared to offer strong support for the social drift hypothesis.

However, Goldberg and Morrison recognised that whilst they seemed to have demonstrated that social drift occurs in association with schizophrenia, their method could not cast any light on the process by which this had occurred. The social class of the patients' fathers was recorded 20–34 years before the patients' current SEC was recorded. The method could not distinguish whether it was the patient or their father who had experienced a social decline. If the parental generation had drifted down the social scale, it might have been a causal factor for their children to develop schizophrenia. This would not constitute social drift. Instead it would reflect social selection into a low SEC of those at risk of schizophrenia. The 'clinical arm' of the study was intended to tease out these possibilities.

A sample of about 80 consecutively admitted men aged 15–29 with an agreed clinical diagnosis of 'definite schizophrenia' were subject to very close history gathering. Hospital and school records were examined. Parents were interviewed and occupational histories were obtained for each extended family. The findings were similar to the 'documentary' arm of the study. The patients' fathers showed a distribution of SEC similar to that for the local area. The patients' distribution of SEC was skewed towards SEC V. Furthermore, when paternal work histories were examined longitudinally, the majority of fathers had experienced an improvement in social position in the patient's lifetime. This social mobility was markedly less for fathers living in the more socially deprived of the two areas studied.

Findings for fathers were broadly reflected in the findings for other relatives, who were said to match the social characteristics of the general population in the areas where they lived. Finally, the patients' school attainment was as good as, or better than, their brothers'. However, their brothers were functioning at a higher occupational level in adulthood. A number of the patients were found to have experienced a sharp occupational decline in the period immediately prior to their first admission to mental hospital. On follow up, the whole sample of patients showed a continuing occupational decline as their illness progressed. There is brief mention of a comparison sample of patients diagnosed as 'definitely not schizophrenic', who were said to have experienced little or no comparable social decline.

Goldberg and Morrison's study is impressive, and it is not surprising that their conclusion *'These findings suggest that gross socio-economic deprivation is unlikely to be of aetiological significance in schizophrenia'* (page 802) was widely accepted. Indeed, the evidence appeared to be so unequivocal that for decades no one felt it was worth replicating the study. However, whilst it is likely that both social selection and social drift do occur, more recent work strongly suggests that the rejection of a causal role for social deprivation in schizophrenia was premature. The contradiction between Goldberg and Morrison's findings and more recent findings may, in part, be due to an assumption that drift down the social gradient and drift into urban areas amount to the same thing. Goldberg and Morrison may have demonstrated social decline following the onset of schizophrenia, but they did not demonstrate that people who were mentally ill moved into inner-city areas as a consequence.

A much more recent Australian study has looked at internal migration from rural areas of people with physical and mental health problems (Moorina *et al.*, 2006). There was no evidence of migration of people with physical health problems from rural areas into cities. In fact, physically ill people migrated to cities less than the healthy population did. There was increased migration from rural areas into cities by people with mental illness, but only small numbers were involved. The authors of the paper speculated that migration might be related to the fact that inpatient facilities were exclusively located in urban settings. The urban drift might therefore be an artefact of the particular social geography of Australia, where there is an exceptionally high degree of urban centralisation of services of all sorts. Furthermore, people admitted to centralised facilities may be discharged to the surrounding area to facilitate follow up.

The Australian study illustrates that a simple assumption that social decline and urban drift go hand in hand may not be valid. It appears self-evident that chronic health problems are likely to have adverse effects on people's income and economic productivity. Goldberg and Morrison's finding of social decline in people diagnosed with schizophrenia may reflect a more profound deleterious effect of being diagnosed with that particular disorder. However, social decline does not automatically lead people to move to inner cities where the incidence of schizophrenia is especially high. Families tend to look after their sick relatives. They tend to work hard to keep them nearby. A large proportion of all people with schizophrenia would have to migrate into inner cities ('urban drift') in order to produce a systematic and substantially higher prevalence in those areas.

Deprivation and utilisation of mental health services

In the UK, health care is largely funded by the state. In the past there have been significant efforts to match levels of funding for services to levels of need in different areas. Attempting to achieve this was ambitious. Imperfect proxy measures had to be used. 'Need' is generally modelled by measuring utilisation of services, and there are factors other than the prevalence of mental disorder in the local population that influence this. For example, it might be that depression is more readily identified and treated in middle-class areas than in deprived inner-city areas for reasons of education, culture or expectation. Similarly, in order to produce a model that would predict need, social deprivation had to be measured through centrally collected data that covered the entire population. This usually meant the national census, which is conducted every ten years.

Glover and colleagues developed such a model in order to guide the rational distribution of resources across different areas (Glover *et al.*, 1998). Centrally collated service utilisation data were compared to measures of social disadvantage from the 1991 UK census using regression analyses. Different population factors predicted admission rates in rural and urban areas. A number of different variables were used in an effort to overcome this, in order to generate a single index, usable across the whole country. The index was calculated from the proportion of adults who were single, widowed or divorced (a measure of social isolation), or lacked access to a car (a measure of poverty), or who were permanently sick or unemployed, or lived in households which were not self-contained, or were staying in boarding houses, hostels or hotels on the census night. As this information was available for every electoral ward in the UK, it could be used to generate a Mental Illness Needs Index (MINI) score for each ward.

The MINI score has been shown to model mental illness need more accurately than other health need indexes, such as the widely used Jarman Underprivileged Area score (Jarman, 1984). The national average MINI score was set as 100. A severely deprived inner-city area might have a score in excess of 135; a wealthy area might have a score under 80. The intention to use MINI scores to rationalise the distribution of resources was never achieved to any great extent. It was one thing to identify those impoverished areas where the need was likely to be greatest. It was quite another to take resources from wealthier areas (with an articulate and politically astute population) and move them to poorer areas. In any case, MINI did not model need perfectly, as was acknowledged by its designers.

Firstly, although MINI scores predicted high levels of need in very deprived areas, the index tended to underestimate the extent of need in those areas. This may be due to flaws in the modelling of demand, or it may be that the relationship between deprivation and the prevalence of mental illness is not linear, or both (Croudace *et al.*, 2000). There are good reasons to suppose that deprivation is not a single continuously distributed variable. It may be that there is a specific type of inner-city deprivation that has a large impact on rates of serious mental illness. MINI may also underestimate need in areas with very low scores, owing to relatively high rates of use of private sector psychiatric services, which would tend to make some need invisible within centrally collated statistics.

Secondly, the effect of a rising MINI score is uneven across different types of mental health problem. Glover and colleagues (Glover *et al.*, 1999) compared the effect of MINI score (and two other mental health need indices) on three different levels of mental health need. These levels of need were aggregated by the type of service that the person used: 'primary care level' need, 'general secondary mental health care level' need and 'forensic mental health care level' need, each level being taken to represent a step up in the severity of mental disorder. The study was primarily concerned with the distribution of resources between services. Despite some acknowledged problems in the data, this mainly statistical study did convincingly show that deprivation had a larger impact on utilisation of forensic secure services than on general psychiatric services, and, somewhat less convincingly, that deprivation had a larger impact on demand for secondary care services than primary care services. There are a number of different ways of interpreting the findings. It might be that offenders or people prone to behavioural disturbance drift into deprived areas. It might be that the effect of social deprivation is to make people more aggressive, and therefore in need of higher levels of care when they become mentally unwell. It might be that deprivation has a causal role in severe mental disorder, but not in less severe illnesses. Any or all of these may be true.

Causation cannot be determined through studies of service utilisation. Nonetheless, they do demonstrate the consistent association between deprivation (especially in inner-city environments) and the most disabling forms of mental illness. Furthermore, the MINI score and its updates have been shown to have a strong correlation with not just service utilisation, but also with prevalence of both psychosis (Croudace *et al.*, 2000), as measured through numbers diagnosed rather than numbers admitted, and common mental disorders as measured in a community survey (Fone *et al.*, 2007).

It seems that deprivation has an impact on a wide range of mental disorders, with a larger effect on more severe disorder. It is unlikely that this is mainly due to a difference in the proportion of people with these disorders who present for treatment in different localities. The deprivation effect is large and consistent in the face of considerable differences in patterns and levels of service provision across geographical areas.

From the 1980s there was a strong (though not universal) psychiatric consensus that schizophrenia is a brain disease, predominantly associated with genetic risk factors. Social risk factors for developing the disorder tended to be regarded as stressors that provoke an illness that has biological causes. Causation is always difficult to firmly establish for mental illnesses, but there is a growing body of evidence that indicates a causal role for social factors. It would be wrong to claim that it is firmly established that schizophrenia is predominantly caused by social adversity. However, there is a realistic possibility that this is the case.

Growing up in the inner city

The reawakening of interest in the nature of the effect of social factors in schizophrenia in recent years has arisen in part from the controversies over the much higher rate of schizophrenia amongst people in the UK whose parents (or grandparents) migrated from the Caribbean (Harrison et al., 1999). This has led researchers to examine the impact of social environment in an increasingly sophisticated way, whereby ethnicity, migration and deprivation have been disaggregated. For example, a well-conducted study from the Institute of Psychiatry confirmed previous findings that when the morbid risk for relatives of White and African–Caribbean people suffering from schizophrenia were compared, first-generation migrants did not differ from the rest of the UK population (Hutchinson et al., 1996). However, the siblings of second-generation migrants with a diagnosis of schizophrenia had a morbid risk seven times as high as their White counterparts. The finding had a high statistical significance.

The likeliest explanation for this startling finding is that second-generation migrants are exposed to an environmental factor that has a massive effect on their risk of developing schizophrenia. The biggest difference between first-generation migrants and their offspring is the location where they spent their childhood. There is further evidence for a strong social factor in the high risk of schizophrenia amongst British Black people. It appears that the impact of being a second-generation African–Caribbean growing up in the UK is greatest in those areas where Black and Ethnic Minority people comprise a smaller proportion of the total population (Kirkbride et al., 2007). In other words, living in areas with a high proportion of people of the same ethnicity appears to confer a degree of protection against the risk associated with being a Black person who has grown up in the UK. None of these findings are easily reconciled with the idea that schizophrenia is primarily caused by genetic factors.

There have been important studies that have examined the effect of social deprivation during childhood. Harrison and colleagues conducted a simple but convincing study in Nottingham as part of a larger project on first-episode psychosis (Harrison et al., 2001a). The participants were 82 people with a research diagnosis of either 'broadly defined schizophrenia' or 'non-schizophrenic psychotic illness' who were born in Nottingham and still lived there. Their birth certificates were obtained, from which was recorded their father's SEC at the time of their birth, and their mother's address. From birth records, 198 controls were identified, matched to the cases for gender, date of birth and area of birth registration.

In the 1970s, Nottingham City Council had developed an index of need within the city, based on 1971 census data. This index was taken as a measure of social deprivation. As 1971 was the median year of birth, it is reasonable to suppose that the score on the index for the mother's address indicated the level of deprivation of the area during the participant's childhood.

For the purpose of the study, areas of Nottingham were divided into two groups; above or below average level of deprivation. This was then combined with paternal SEC at birth to create a three-level childhood deprivation score:

- 0 if father was social class I–III and mother lived in a non-deprived area.
- 1 if father was social class IV–V *or* mother lived in a deprived area
- 2 if father was social class IV–V *and* mother lived in a deprived area

There was a consistent association of adult-onset psychosis with paternal social class and area level deprivation. However, the combined childhood deprivation score showed a highly significant linear association with all psychoses and with broad schizophrenia. The association for non-schizophrenic psychosis was weaker. The size of the effect was substantial. People over 25 years who had a childhood deprivation score of 2 were much more likely to suffer from broad schizophrenia as those with a score of 0.

The Harrison study attempted to control for possible confounding factors, including ethnicity, family history, and drift into deprived areas (to exclude social drift or selection or segregation effects). Controlling for African–Caribbean ethnicity did reduce the size of the effect somewhat, but it remained large. The study, though lacking methodological sophistication and sufficient statistical power to answer all the relevant questions, stands in contradiction to the Goldberg and Morrison work on social drift. Here we have striking evidence suggesting that the social environment you grow up in has a profound effect on the chances of developing a major mental illness in adulthood.

There have been very long-standing suspicions that city life might be bad for your mental health, with a history stretching back to the nineteenth century. Until recently the evidence with regard to the differential effects of urban and rural poverty has been equivocal. Some ambiguity remains (particularly concerning disorders other than schizophrenia), but the weight of evidence is that growing up in urban deprivation has a particularly toxic effect. A systematic review of the literature between 1950 and 2009 on factors affecting the incidence of schizophrenia in England found that the relationship with urbanicity was one of the few consistent findings (Kirkbride *et al.*, 2012a).

A credible study has suggested that the considerable difference in the number of people with schizophrenia using services in rural Dumfries and Galloway and urban Camberwell (61% higher in Camberwell) might be entirely due to the presence in Camberwell of a large non-White population with a high risk of mental illness (Allardyce *et al.*, 2001). The White populations in the two locations had similar rates of schizophrenia. This finding runs against most of the evidence (for example, the Nottingham study cited above). The authors point out that excluding the non-White population from the Camberwell sample in order to calculate prevalence in a White sub-sample may well have disproportionately eliminated people with lower social class. An American study has suggested that the urbanicity effect on the prevalence of schizophrenia has been evident since at least 1880 (Torrey & Bowler, 1990). Cities have always grown through migration, but this has often been due to a movement of the rural population within a nation. It is difficult to reconcile the persistence of the epidemiological pattern with the idea that the excess of people with a diagnosis of schizophrenia in urban areas is an artefact of the number of offspring of migrants from overseas living there.

Perhaps the most important evidence that early exposure to urban deprivation has an association with later mental illness, at least with respect to schizophrenia, comes from cohort studies. These are mostly based on Scandinavian record systems which allow data linkage in large populations. A Swedish cohort of 49,000 national service conscripts has been much studied, as medical and psychiatric evaluations on conscription aged 18 years could be linked to later health records. Findings from a study on this cohort showed an incidence of schizophrenia 1.65 times higher in those who grew up in cities compared to those who had a rural childhood (Lewis *et al.*, 1992).

A study of the whole Swedish population aged 25–65 years found a relationship between population density and risk of mental illness. Those living in the most densely populated areas had 68–77% more risk of developing psychosis and 12–20% more risk of developing severe depression leading to hospital admission (Sundquist *et al.*, 2004).

The most compelling evidence on urbanicity is a Danish population study showing a dose–response effect (Pedersen & Mortensen, 2001). The greater the number of years that individuals were exposed to an urban environment before their 15th birthday, whether continuously or intermittently, the higher the risk of developing schizophrenia later. Furthermore, the intensity of the urban environment also had an effect.

The toxic factor

Although there are some contradictions within the literature, it is quite certain that rates of diagnosis of mental illness of most types are higher amongst poor people than the rest of the population. In addition to this, it seems that there is a special association between inner-city deprivation in childhood and adult schizophrenia. To find firm evidence of social antecedents for a mental illness that has been so widely regarded as having a biological basis is contrary to expectation. Despite the strength of the evidence, it is possible that the effect of urban deprivation may yet prove to be due to some unknown confounding factor. This seems unlikely to us. Urban deprivation can be regarded as an established causal factor. It is worth considering what the nature of the toxic factor in a deprived urban childhood might be. This is explored in detail in Chapter 7. There is an important question to ask at this stage concerning inequality as opposed to poverty per se.

Wilkinson and Pickett (2009) have demonstrated that for the developed world within-country income inequality correlates more closely to health and social problems in the population than absolute poverty. Their findings suggested that local inequalities are less important than overall national inequalities. They have been criticised for giving the impression that they identified an invariable rule applicable to all health and social problems. The suggestion is that they reify interesting findings into a general law of health inequality (Muller, 2002; Mackenbach, 2002; Osler *et al.*, 2002).

The role of social factors in schizophrenia appears to contradict this, as local income inequality may be important. In trying to understand what might be unusual about inner-city areas other than the absolute level of deprivation, the existence of marked local inequalities is immediately evident as a candidate factor. Deprived inner-city areas are located close to more prosperous areas. Wealthy inner-city areas are amongst the most privileged of social environments. The consequence of the close juxtaposition of the poorest and wealthiest urban areas is that the inner-city population are constantly confronted with the extent of their disadvantage and with their exclusion from a much better life. Their noses are pressed against the shop window, but there is no way of gaining entry to the store.

A handful of well-conducted studies have examined the effect of local inequalities on the prevalence of psychosis. Whilst the findings are not conclusive, they are interesting. Boydell and colleagues (Boydell *et al.*, 2004a) conducted a retrospective case note study of individuals presenting with first-onset schizophrenia using Research Diagnostic Criteria (RDC) in Camberwell, London, analysing the findings by electoral ward. They found that whilst there was no overall association between incidence and inequality, where the level of deprivation was highest, there was an effect due to the level of local inequality. This persisted after adjustment for a range of factors, including those related to ethnicity. In other words, there was an increased incidence of schizophrenia in those deprived electoral wards that also had the highest levels of inequality. The effect was substantial (Incidence Rate Ratio = 3.79, p = 0.019). This is compatible with the suggestion that there are specific social environments that are associated with unusually high rates of schizophrenia, and that these environments are characterised by both high levels of deprivation and high levels of inequality. This might look suspiciously like a specific pathogenic environment.

Burns and Esterhuizen (2008) reported a similar study from South Africa that used a less complex measure of inequality. They found that poverty alone did not affect the incidence of schizophrenia, but that income inequality did, and that this held true after adjusting for urbanicity. Clearly there are many differences between South Africa and the UK, but local inequality seems to have a particularly toxic effect in both environments. Furthermore, the finding that local inequality has an effect independent of urbanicity would tend to support the idea that the toxicity of inner cities is mediated by high levels of local inequality.

On the basis of another very large study using Swedish data linkage systems, Zammit and colleagues (Zammit *et al.*, 2010) have suggested that the effect of urbanicity is mediated by what they call 'social fragmentation'. Essentially this is an index that combines a variety of measures of locality level social instability. There is little doubt that the phenomena that they group together under the rubric 'social fragmentation' are present in the areas with the highest incidence of schizophrenia. It is more difficult to know if these are the factors that actually influence the development of schizophrenia. However, the same can be said of income inequality. Whilst a variety of social circumstances may *characterise* the environments that are particularly schizophrenogenic, there is nothing to support or refute the suggestion that they are essential parts of a causal chain between the social environment and the development of schizophrenia in individuals.

Two types of model

In looking for mechanisms mediating between social factors and mental illness, there are two overarching approaches: *reductive* theories that suggest chains of causation through specific and individually measurable factors, and *emergence* theories that suggest a specific and irreducible effect that arises when a critical mass of specific factors come together to have an impact that is greater than the sum of the parts. We will return to these two models in several subsequent chapters.

Using a reductive approach, there have been efforts to develop theories linking migrant status, inner-city childhood, psychological consequences and brain mechanisms that are known to have a relationship with psychotic symptoms (broadly speaking neuronal circuits mediated by dopamine that control arousal). Many of these theories invoke the psychological concept of social defeat (Selten & Cantor-Graae, 2005). Social defeat is a chronic sense of being a social outsider with subordinate status. It is associated with an inability to influence one's own circumstances or to secure those material circumstances and possessions that are generally accepted to be the trappings of success and well-being. Social defeat has been shown to be more prevalent amongst populations at high risk for developing mental illness (Stowkowy & Addington, 2012). This is an essentially reductionist model that invokes known mechanisms, but creates a causal chain of uncertain validity. These ideas are explored more fully in Chapter 7.

The emergence view is that increasing social adversity has a cumulative effect in making life more difficult and stressful, but there is a critical mass of social adversity where all aspects of life become so difficult that there is a stepwise leap in adverse effects. This view understands the inner-city effect on the incidence of schizophrenia as an emergent phenomenon, requiring various elements, but not reducible to any specific factor or simple addition of multiple factors. A much greater than additive effect emerges once a critical level of social adversity is reached. It has been suggested that this may arise where early adversity creates circumstances that beget cumulative later adversity, with a cascade of catastrophic social disadvantage (Morgan & Hutchinson, 2010). This too is explored in Chapter 7.

Is incidence changing over time?

Two of the key tests of the validity of a scientific theory are that it should both explain what is known and predict future findings. If specific social environments cause schizophrenia, then changes in social environments should alter the incidence of the disorder over time. Cities exist in a state of continuous change and development. Some areas deteriorate whilst others become fashionable and desirable. Industries spring up or disappear. Populations move in response to changes in the demand for labour. British income inequality was relatively low from the end of the Second World War until 1980, since when it has steadily increased to levels that are very high compared with other developed countries.[1] The social environment in the inner cities has deteriorated substantially during this time. Both local inequality and social fragmentation have increased. If growing up in these particular social conditions is a potent cause of schizophrenia, then one would expect evidence of an increase in the incidence of the disorder. The peak of African-Caribbean migration to the UK occurred in the 1950s and 1960s. Two further generations have been born in this country, and the proportion of the population with such a background has grown. This could also be expected to lead to an increase in the incidence of schizophrenia.

Examination of UK administrative figures appears to suggest that the incidence of psychosis, and particularly schizophrenia, dropped in the course of the twentieth century. However, the systematic review of incidence figures reported in studies spanning a 60-year period is equivocal (Kirkbride *et al.*, 2012a). Some studies suggest a drop in incidence since the Second World War and some suggest an increase. Studies in Camberwell (for example, Alladyce *et al.*, 2001) definitely suggest an increase, but this has occurred against the backdrop of major demographic change in that area. Given the apparent strength of the evidence for social causation of schizophrenia, it is troubling to find that the evidence on changes in national incidence is ambiguous. There are a variety of ways of explaining this apparent paradox. They include the possibility that there are different forces at play with opposing effects of unequal strength. Some tend to reduce incidence and others increase it. The combined impact has different effects in different locations, creating an ambiguous overall picture.

This may give the impression that a firmly predicted change in incidence has not arisen in response to observed changes in inequality. However, we do not know the exact nature of the toxic factor. Economic inequality in the UK has worsened,

---

[1] Organisation for Economic Co-operation and Development (2011) *Divided We Stand: Why Inequality Keeps Rising.* www.oecd.org/els/social/inequality *retrieved 18 March 2013.*

but this does not necessarily mean that a larger proportion of British children have been exposed to the social conditions that have a specific adverse effect on future mental health. Whilst we know how many children grow up in poverty, we don't know how many of these grow up in the most toxic type of poverty. It is more the case that there is a gap in the evidence rather than true contradictions. Whilst the arguments for a major role for social causation of schizophrenia are strong and compelling, we cannot tie observed changes in social environment to predicted changes in incidence. This is a problem.

What about bipolar affective disorder?

Whilst the relationship between urban deprivation and schizophrenia is well established, the same cannot be said for bipolar affective disorder. There have been far fewer studies of risk factors in bipolar affective disorder than in schizophrenia. The evidence that exists mainly comes from studies whose primary focus is schizophrenia. Since the 1930s, these studies have shown that the impact of urbanicity on the incidence of bipolar affective disorder is less than for schizophrenia. Some studies show a similar but attenuated urban effect on bipolar affective disorder. Some show that urbanicity has no effect for this disorder. A modern Danish data linkage study has shown a weak effect of urbanicity (Mortensen *et al.*, 2003). A prospective study from Ireland suggests that the incidence of bipolar affective disorder may be higher in rural areas than in urban areas (Kelly *et al.*, 2010). In this study, the Incidence Rate Ratio (IRR) for schizophrenia in urban areas vs. rural areas was 1.92 for men and 1.34 for women. For affective psychosis the IRR for men was 0.48 for men and 0.60 for women. In other words, urbanicity had opposite effects in the two disorders.

It is hard to know what to make of these findings. There is no reason why bipolar affective disorder should have similar social origins to schizophrenia if they are distinct syndromes. However, there is some evidence that they may not be separate disorders at all. The Danish linkage study mentioned above showed that a family history of schizophrenia was a risk factor for bipolar affective disorder. It has been recognised for a very long time that many people present with psychotic symptoms that are a mixture of the two, so-called schizoaffective disorder. Some research into the genetics of mental disorder suggests that they are not separate conditions, and there are differences in opinion over how this might work genetically (Crow, 2008; Craddock & Owen, 2007). This kind of evidence that invokes a unitary psychosis instead of two distinct disorders is difficult to reconcile with the evidence on childhood social factors.

Conclusion

We have examined only a fraction of the literature here, but the broad outline of the relationship between social inequality and mental illness is evident. Mental illness tends to be commoner amongst people with low incomes, and nearly all mental illnesses have an association with social adversity. The association appears to be strongest for schizophrenia.

There are two factors relating to childhood that have a potent effect in increasing the risk of developing schizophrenia as an adult. One is ethnicity. The other is deprived urban environment. There are inconsistencies in the evidence, and some puzzling findings, but growing up in urban deprivation, and facing adversity related to ethnicity, appear to be credible as major causal factors in schizophrenia (Van Os, 2004). The implications of this are only just beginning to be seen in the psychiatric literature.

Main points in this chapter

1. There have been consistent research findings showing higher rates of schizophrenia amongst poorer people.
2. There are particularly high rates of schizophrenia amongst people exposed to urban deprivation in childhood. The greater the exposure, the higher the risk.
3. The evidence for an association between urban poverty and bipolar affective disorder is far weaker and the association may be non-existent. This is puzzling in the face of evidence that the two conditions are closely related to each other.
4. It is reasonable to believe that social factors have a causal role in schizophrenia.
5. There are significant contradictions in the evidence that cannot easily be explained. There are also major gaps in the evidential chain.
6. It is impossible to choose between a *reductive* model where many separate factors come together to make urban environments schizophrenogenic and an *emergence* model where a set of specific social characteristics lead to a powerful unitary pathogenic effect.

2

Poverty

Britain has one of the largest economies in the world, and this status has not been changed by an extended economic depression. Its major cities do not have shanty town slums, such as can be seen in Mumbai or Rio De Janeiro. Manifest severe poverty is so uncommon in the UK that the British visitor to the USA is shocked at the sight of large impoverished neighbourhoods on the outskirts of American conurbations. Essential health care remains mostly free at the point of delivery in the UK, and there is access to food and shelter for even the poorest, provided they are able to seek it out.

Explicit discussion of poverty has returned to British public life in the context of a persistent global financial crisis that has led to significant reductions in income for all but the wealthiest part of the population. Prior to the onset of the banking crisis in 2007, there was a mainstream political consensus that a long and unbroken period of economic growth had raised living standards to such an extent that the concept of domestic poverty was outmoded and no longer applicable to the UK population. Poverty was now something that happened in Africa. However, even during the long economic boom that started in the 1990s, there were growing problems for the section of the UK population with the lowest income. Firstly, the gap between their income and the income of the richest part of the population was widening. Secondly, their income was not increasing. In fact, after adjustment for inflation, their income was dropping.[1] Not only were they becoming poorer in relative terms, they were becoming poorer in absolute terms. The political belief that wealth would 'trickle down' as national income increased had proven false. The onset of the present economic depression significantly increased the existing trend towards greater social inequality. Although similar changes are evident in comparable European countries, these changes are most marked in the UK (Hills, 2010).

---

[1] Brewer M, Goodman A, Muriel A, Sibieta L (2007) *Poverty and inequality in the UK 2007* IFFS Briefing Note 73, The Institute for Fiscal Studies www.ifss.org.uk/bns/bn73.pdf *retrieved 6 September 2012.*

Whilst the everyday use of the term poverty may appear uncomplicated, describing poverty in a scientific and robust way is difficult. There are layers of complexity, as poverty extends beyond a simple lack of material resource. *Absolute poverty* implies a lack of the means to secure fundamental human needs such as food, shelter, water, sanitation, basic education and so on. There is no substantial part of the UK population living with this type of poverty at present, although small numbers of people are in want of basic necessities. For the most part, in the Western world, poverty means a lack of resources compared to other people, *relative poverty*. There are a number of different ways of thinking about this, all of which have limitations.

Income

Monetary income is the simplest measure of poverty or wealth in a developed economy. However, it is necessary to take into account the impact of direct and indirect taxation in order to arrive at an estimate of net income. In agrarian societies, some necessities are secured without exchanging money. For example, villagers may join together to use their collective labour to harvest crops. There are few examples of economic community collectivism in the UK, although there are some co-operative ventures organised at a local level, such as skill exchanges.

In making comparisons between countries or over time, differences in costs of commodities are important. For example, the cost of accommodation, food and public transport relative to each other can change or differ, making some necessities easier to secure than others. New commodities are developed and these can come to be understood to be necessities. Computers and mobile phones are examples. Over time a family has to use a higher proportion of its income on accommodation, but they can now afford computers and mobile phones. Have they become richer or poorer?

Income is difficult to measure and the purchasing power of income changes over short time spans. In any case, income has little meaning unless it is compared with the income of other groups or the whole of society.

Inequality

There is a variety of methods of measuring inequality, and there are different types of inequality. For example, if incomes are divided into centiles, the top and bottom centiles can have particularly high and low incomes (and therefore high levels of inequality), whilst differences between the other eight centiles can be relatively small (a sigmoid distribution). This is different from more evenly spaced income differences between consecutive centiles on a steep gradient (a linear distribution).

The measure of income inequality most commonly used by economists is the Gini co-efficient. This is a statistical measure of inequality among values in frequency distributions. There are some problems with applying it to income, and there are several different ways of adjusting the calculation. Nonetheless, it is the generally accepted way of measuring and comparing income inequality. A Gini co-efficient value of 0 means absolute equality (i.e. no variation in income between individuals) and 1 means absolute inequality (i.e. one individual gets all the income and everybody else has none). In comparisons of inequality between developed nations, Gini co-efficients vary between 0.30 and 0.55. When making comparisons of the health impact of inequality between nations, cruder measures of inequality (for example, the ratio of income of the top 20% and bottom 20%) produce similar results. Whether measures are sophisticated or crude, there is strong evidence that inequality affects health and well-being.

In 2009, Wilkinson and Pickett summarised the evidence about the health and social consequences of income inequality in a book called *The Spirit Level* (Wilkinson & Pickett, 2009). Much of the evidence comes from their own research. The book has made a significant impact well beyond the academic community. It has fuelled debate across the political spectrum. It describes a consistent pattern whereby a wide range of social and health problems are more prevalent in developed economies where there are higher levels of income inequality. There is no consistent pattern between these countries related to unadjusted per capita income. Wilkinson and Pickett illustrate this with respect to life expectancy, violence, teenage pregnancy, drug use, obesity and a range of other problems, including depression and social mobility. The implications seem clear. In some important way it is worse for you to be poor when income inequality is large than where it is small, irrespective of absolute income.

Although Wilkinson and Pickett go to some lengths to emphasise that the ideas in the book are based on empirical data from independent sources, and upon peer-reviewed research reports, they are unapologetic in promoting greater equality as a solution to public health problems. This has obvious political implications, and it is not surprising to find that their work has come under fierce and sustained attack, mainly from the political right (e.g. Snowdon, 2010). They have been accused of manipulating statistics and of misconstruing other authors' work. Wilkinson and Pickett make a key argument that societies that are more equal are better places for everyone, including the rich. In making this point they are accused of conflating an adverse impact of inequality on disadvantaged individuals with an adverse impact on society as a whole.

Wilkinson and Pickett have robustly defended their work. In particular, they have denied a partisan political motive. They have rejected the suggestion that they believe that they have identified an invariable 'law of inequality' that accounts for all differences in rates of social and health problems. Instead, they claim to have demonstrated a general pattern. Although there are significant exceptions, the pattern recurs surprisingly frequently, and with an effect size that would tend to support a causal role for inequality in a wide range of problems.

The literature setting out the controversies over *The Spirit Level* can be accessed easily[2] and readers can make up their own minds over the balance of the evidence. In our opinion, the research cited and conclusions reached by Wilkinson and Pickett do withstand critical scrutiny, and their general point is not undermined by the fact that the pattern they describe is not invariable. For example, they observe that *in general* it is inequalities at a regional or national scale that matter. This does not hold true in the *particular case* of schizophrenia and urban childhood, where the evidence tends to suggest that local inequalities may be important (see Chapter 1). There is no reason why social inequality at a regional or national level should have the same effect on every disorder or upon different mental disorders such as bipolar affective disorder compared with schizophrenia. There is no contradiction or inconsistency between the two.

Social class

Historically, social class has been one of the main ways that politicians and social scientists have understood the structure of society. More recently, British politicians have eliminated the use of terminology relating to class from political discourse, which reflects a new reluctance amongst the two main parliamentary parties to portray themselves as representatives of distinct class interests. Both prefer to construe themselves as representing '*middle England*'. This is an evidently imaginary construct that is routinely invoked as a national archetype. John Major used it in a positive way when he was Prime Minister, '*the country of long shadows on cricket grounds, warm beer, invincible green suburbs, dog lovers and pools fillers, and, as George Orwell said, "Old maids bicycling to holy communion through the morning mist"*'.[3] It has also been used as an insult. Napoleon Bonaparte quoted Adam Smith: '*a nation of shopkeepers*'.

It is unlikely that a significant proportion of the UK population match either characterisation. Although the proportion of people that regard themselves as having any social class at all has declined, in 2010 over a third of the population saw the concept of class as relevant to them (Savage *et al.*, 2010). There is an important sub-cultural element to class that can be highly idiosyncratic to particular countries, and serves to perpetuate the segregation of social groups. For example, the South Asian construct of caste has proven surprisingly robust in the face of major political, economic and social change. Whilst it would be wrong to say that efforts to eliminate it have failed completely, caste remains a salient concept. It has a continuing impact on people's lives.

Similarly, class has a particular relevance and meaning to White Britons. Classifications of socio-economic class (SEC) and proxies such as highest educational

---

[2] http://www.equalitytrust.org.uk *retrieved 28 May 2013*.
[3] Speech to the Conservative Group for Europe, 22 April 1993.

attainment are crude measures, and they completely fail to capture the idiosyncratic British construct of class. Class is as much a cultural point of reference as it is a descriptor of income or lifestyle. Where socially mobile Americans are generally keen to identify themselves as 'middle class', things are different in the UK. Socially mobile Britons who are objectively well educated and wealthy can regard themselves as 'working class' because their parents or their grandparents were manual workers. This may reflect an inverted snobbery, whereby it is better to be seen to have achieved in the face of adversity than to have achieved on the basis of privilege.

Two hundred years ago the Industrial Revolution was accompanied by huge changes in British society, both social and intellectual. Large numbers of agricultural workers migrated to cities to find employment in new industries. The Enlightenment and rationalism affected all types of intellectual endeavour, including the formation of new disciplines of economics, sociology and psychiatry. Politicians increasingly attempted to justify themselves by reference to scientific theories and evidence. Structural ways of understanding and describing social class became popular at this time.

Marx and Engels drew on the old approach of philosophy and on new ideas that would become sociology and economics to justify their radical socialism. They defined social class in terms of the relationship of the individual to the means of production (Marx & Engels, 2008). According to them, under capitalism there are two main classes, the bourgeoisie, who own and control capital, and the proletariat, workers in industry who must sell their labour to survive. Other classes (for example, the petit bourgeois, peasantry, and intelligentsia) are essentially irrelevant, as it is the conflict of economic interest between the bourgeoisie and the proletariat that drives turbulence and social progress in capitalist society. This way of understanding society and economics has been highly influential on both the left and the right. It is a way of analysing social divisions that has survived the discrediting effects of the realities of communist regimes. As a way of understanding the fine grain of social status and difference, conceptualising social class solely on the basis of economic relationships and class struggle is simplistic. It is of limited value in understanding the impact of deprivation on individuals.

Max Weber was one of the nineteenth-century founders of the social sciences alongside Marx and Durkheim. Like Marx he was politically active on the left. Weber took the view that Marx's model of social class was too narrow and lacked social meaning. He had a broader model of structural relationships within society, whereby social class was one aspect of social stratification. Social stratification, according to Weber, has three inter-related elements: economic status, social status and power (Käsler, 1989). His model was sophisticated and sufficiently flexible to accommodate to social changes such as alterations in the relative kudos of different occupations over time.

Weber's ideas had some influence when administrative class categorisations started to be developed in order to understand troubling phenomena such as big variations in perinatal and childhood mortality rates in different geographical

---

Box 1 National Statistics Socio-economic Classification (NS-SEC)

Class 1. Higher managerial and professional occupations
        1.1 Large employers and high managerial occupations
        1.2 Higher professional occupations
Class 2. Lower managerial and professional occupations
Class 3. Intermediate occupations
Class 4. Small employers and own-account workers
Class 5. Lower supervisory and technical occupations
Class 6. Semi-routine occupations
Class 7. Routine occupations
Class 8. Never worked and long-term unemployed

---

areas. In 1913 a categorisation of SEC was developed in the UK by the Registrar General's Office (Szreter, 1984). Versions of it remained in use until 2001. The system identified six social classes (or socio-economic groups, SEGs), I to VI, where VI was 'Other'. The system was based on the level of skill required to work in each occupation. SEG I was 'professional' and included, for example, doctors; SEG V was 'unskilled manual workers', who represented a large proportion of the population when the classification was devised, but which has subsequently declined numerically through the effects of mechanisation and globalisation.

The hierarchy reflected the social status of various occupations. In a 1951 revision, SEG III was divided into IIIa (skilled, non-manual) and IIIb (skilled, manual). In 2001, the Office for National Statistics developed a new classification, the National Statistics Socio-Economic Classification (NS-SEC) which replaced the existing systems for identifying occupational or social groups in the population. It is related to a research classification and comprises eight classes (see Box 1) (Walthery, 2006).

As a general approach, understanding social class by occupation has its problems. For example, some occupations, such as 'farmer', include a very wide range of incomes and levels of property ownership. Finding meaningful boundaries between, for example, smallholders and aristocratic landowners is not easy. Nonetheless this approach to understanding social stratification has persisted for 100 years. This is mainly attributable to the fact that consistent differences continue to be evident across the groups, often in the form of a gradient of rates of health and social problems.

Class is a construct that shows little sign of disappearing from the social sciences literature, despite a gradual decrease in its social and political salience. There might be three main reasons for its persistence.

Firstly, social class might be an artefact of different ways of aggregating and analysing social differences, a useful way of making social phenomena manageable without reflecting real social structures. The belief that you or someone else belong to the 'working class' or 'middle class' might be a cultural construct with no objective reality. By analogy, it is fairly certain that the Freudian 'ego' and 'id' do not exist as objective elements of the human mind, but they continue to be widely referred to as if they do. Psychoanalytic concepts have become part of Western culture, both popular and intellectual. The same may be true of class.

Secondly, and conversely, social classes may exist as real social groupings, whether or not individuals realise that they are part of them. Being born into a particular social class can be seen to have an effect on people's ability to earn money and to achieve, independent of their capabilities. This follows the reasoning of Marx and others. Conflicts in class interests are suggested to be the cause of poverty. The dominant class of capital owners has an intrinsic interest in paying low wages to workers, without making them so poor that they are unable to purchase goods sold to them for profit. Workers are held above penury but below comfort. Class is not always perceived, but has an effect on life regardless.

Finally, social class may be a consequence of differences in ability. Society may be a meritocracy where stratification arises from assortment and ordering according to ability. It might be that people remain in the class they are born into because offspring tend to have abilities similar to those of their parents. The lowest social classes would be seen to exist because, in Western societies, survival of the fittest operates in the absence of a lethal consequence of inferiority. This is the implicit model underlying the concept of the *underclass*, an idea that lacks any clear validation, but which has proven very popular with politicians, the current-affairs media and influential think tanks. We discuss the *underclass* in Chapter 3.

Social capital

Social capital has crept into the language of social policy over the last 30 years, bringing with it something of a conceptual fog. The idea has attracted a lot of attention amongst social theorists, economists and, latterly, politicians. Broadly speaking, 'social capital' comprises non-financial resources and other advantages that can be gained through relationships and networks. It is generally regarded as being distinct from 'cultural capital', which are non-financial assets such as education, knowledge, skills and social standing that are held by individuals and give them an advantage over other people. Social and cultural capital belong mostly to the privileged. They are amongst the perceived advantages of private education. Social capital is not held by the individual, but exists in social networks to which they belong. It arises from relationships and patterns of interaction. Trust and reciprocity are fundamental to social capital. The concept is sometimes reified as if it were measurable or even could be traded like monetary capital. This has led to efforts to enumerate social capital, with assessments of the amount and quality of resources that come in this form to different groups.

There are many sources and consequences of social capital. For example, economists suggest that people who have access to higher levels of social capital are more likely to be in paid employment. There is a circularity here as being in employment creates opportunities to engage with social networks. Social capital has been suggested as a moderating factor in neighbourhoods with high levels of risk factors associated with psychiatric disorders. Differences in levels of social capital might account for varying rates of mental disorder between areas that are otherwise similar. Social capital exists in the structure of social networks. It is accessed by individuals by engaging with other people or organisations. It can be said to have both structural aspects (which affect whole social networks) and cognitive aspects (which affect individuals' self-perception).

One of the explanations for the lack of social capital in deprived urban areas is that intra-neighbourhood relationships are poor, which reduces opportunities to generate new social capital. If one ignores for a moment the tautological nature of this proposition, this might be one of the factors that make living in these areas difficult and stressful. Researchers use a variety of methods to measure social capital. These include social network analysis and direct measurement of the frequency of certain features in the immediate environment, such as graffiti, vandalism, gangs, racism and so on.

Increasing the level of social capital is said to be amenable to social policy intervention at a locality and at a societal level. This is a key point of contention. If lack of social capital is an inevitable consequence of neighbourhood poverty, then interventions that do not address poverty directly are unlikely to be effective. Attempts to reduce poverty by increasing social capital might be similar to trying to cure a disease by treating one of its symptoms in isolation.

It is certainly possible to understand some of the problems of poor people in terms of low social capital, whereby they lack the social connections to improve their situation or to improve the quality of life within their community. Even when the term 'social capital' was first coined, it was not a novel concept. Lack of social capital has echoes of the ideas of Marx, Durkheim and others. Social capital can be understood to include elements of social solidarity, and it can be seen as the opposite of Marx's alienation or Durkheim's anomie. Social capital is usually conceptualised in terms of non-financial resources, but Bourdieu, the most influential social theorist of the 1980s, regarded social capital and economic capital as inseparable (Bourdieu, 1986). Indeed, Bourdieu saw social capital in negative terms. To him, these were the non-financial assets arising from exclusive networks that the middle class and the upper class use to exclude poor people from their social world of privilege.

The intentional destruction of the power of the trade union movement in the 1980s can be understood as a determined effort to undermine or destroy social capital amongst the industrial working class. The current political orthodoxy, accepted by all mainstream British parties, is that the trade unions were 'too strong' in the 1970s, and that it was important for the national interest that steps were taken to reduce their power. However, trade union strength meant that they had the ability to promote the economic interests of the unionised working class. The taming of labour organisations has been associated with increasing social inequalities, and with a loss of the distinctive working-class social organisations associated with the labour movement. Seen in this way, social capital is inextricably linked to class interest. Social capital has a different connotation depending on one's position in the social order.

Whether or not the taming of organised labour through trade union reforms in the 1980s was a good thing, a great deal of working-class social capital was destroyed at this time. The loss of distinctive working-class organisations was an inevitable consequence of the closure of major industries such as steel-making and mining. All manner of social networks, from social clubs and sports facilities to educational and political resources, were lost. This has had a major and enduring impact on large industrial working-class communities, which were predominantly located in the north and west of the UK.

Even in areas where this did not happen, the sale of council houses and the successful development of a 'property-owning democracy' undermined social cohesion in large council estates. Rented municipal housing stock was allowed to physically deteriorate and was increasingly occupied by people with the worst social problems and the weakest financial resources. Their presence in neighbourhoods of mixed rental and owner occupation reduced the market value of privately owned properties. Whether or not these consequences were foreseen, the loss of social capital and social solidarity amongst the poorest section of British society arose directly from government policies designed to fundamentally alter social values and allegiances.

Social and cultural capital have some explanatory power in understanding the relationship between inner-city communities and deviant or marginal counter-cultures, including gangs and other social groupings that are intensely bonded but disconnected from mainstream society. Criminal gangs provide young people, particularly men, with access to social and cultural capital that they cannot otherwise acquire. Established criminal 'families', well known in their neighbourhoods, often straddle legitimate business and criminal activity. They provide a social kinship structure, bonds of loyalty and mutual protection. They often have an ambiguous role in their local community. They can be involved in vigilante policing and maintenance of social order, albeit through the application of some unusual social values backed up with violence. They can deploy a type of pseudo-philanthropy, for example supporting charities or community activities, giving a positive spin to a social standing that is otherwise mainly dependent upon intimidation.

Membership of all types of social networks can have disadvantages as well as advantages, not least because networks always demand conformity to a specific set of values. Formalised networks invariably expect individuals to place the needs of the network itself above narrow personal self-interest. Criminal families and networks are no different in this regard. Some people in inner-city communities live on the edge of both mainstream society and criminal networks. It is difficult to conform to mainstream social values whilst accommodating to close proximity to a criminal sub-culture. This causes major problems as their imperatives are incompatible. For example, the desire to live free from fear of crime cannot be reconciled with an imperative that sees co-operation with the police as a betrayal of the community as a whole.

Inner-city life

Neither absolute nor relative poverty capture the full variety of ways of being poor. Although poverty can be measured as a continuous variable determined by the value of personal assets, it is actually made up of a range of distinct social circumstances. Poverty is characterised as much by the fact that life is difficult as it is by a lack of cash.

Inner-city poverty has particular features that go far beyond a special relationship with major mental illness. For example, rates of car ownership are low in inner cities, and this creates an obstruction to employment. Public transport is expensive. Across the UK, grocery retailing is dominated by large supermarkets. These are organised on the premise that most customers will travel to them in privately owned motor vehicles. They are relatively inaccessible for people in the inner city, who tend to rely on small local shops instead, where goods are expensive because of high overheads. Together with other similar factors, this makes basic necessities more expensive for the inner-city population than it is for middle-class people, which in turn reduces their ability to use their income for anything other than the costs of daily living. Lack of disposable income makes it difficult to access the full range of leisure pursuits and learning opportunities that are available to the rest of the community. In the face of mainstream attitudes that value self-improvement, poor people in inner cities are confronted with seemingly insurmountable barriers to improving their lives.

When community psychiatrists working in inner-city areas visit patients at home, they are sometimes welcomed into an orderly but sparsely furnished sitting room dominated by an incongruously large state-of-the-art television permanently tuned to a subscription channel. People in inner-city poverty tend to perceive themselves as unable to increase their income. Advertisers and retailers constantly confront them with a huge range of luxury consumer goods. High-quality televisions, for example, are available to them but at a much higher true cost than to the rest of the population, as they can only be paid for if other priorities are neglected. Denied access to a full range of diversion and leisure pursuits, home entertainment is often central to their lives. There is comfort in owning a high-prestige item in the face of an otherwise limited life. The paradox of an oversized and expensive item in a small and poverty-stricken household is an incongruity only to the educated professional. The choice looks more rational in the context of a life where progress is unlikely to happen.

People living in inner-city poverty are more frequently victims of crime than wealthier urban dwellers. This is as true for domestic burglary as it is for violent assaults. People in these areas often feel that policing is something that is done to them rather than done for them, and one can understand how they come to feel this (Kusow *et al.*, 1997; Murphy & Cherney, 2012). Some police officers experience themselves as being under attack by these communities. They feel that they are struggling with a population that is, if not intrinsically criminal, then more than usually protective of the criminals in its midst. These conflicting attitudes create long-term tensions that from time to time express themselves as riots, with pitched battles between police and young people.

People in inner-city areas often see themselves as having a double problem with authority, with the police being the most visible element of this. They complain that the police do nothing to protect them from crime and yet persecute them by making assumptions about criminality. They feel that the police regard their community and the individuals within it as uniformly and intrinsically criminal. There is an identifiable set of self-perceptions linked to this. People experience themselves as passive victims in a series of misfortunes. They feel let down or cheated by specific authority figures or by social institutions in general. Although this victimised mind set is understandable, it is dysfunctional as it undermines the sense of agency that is known to be associated with resilience (Summerfield, 2001). It generates a vicious cycle of anger, passivity and further misfortune. It creates a reluctance to accept such help as is available, which is inevitably delivered by authority figures who are expected to prove unreliable.

Rural poverty

Across the world, the vast majority of poor people live in rural environments. In keeping with the rest of the developed world, this is not the case in the UK. However, rural poverty is an important phenomenon, and it differs in a number of ways from urban poverty.

Contemporary rural poverty in the UK was described in some detail in a report for the Commission for Rural Communities that was published in 2009.[4] The report was based upon routinely collected government statistics. Very few indices of poverty or deprivation are worse in rural areas than in urban areas. Generally speaking, the prevalence of poverty is either similar in rural areas to urban areas, or somewhat less in rural areas. This is seen, for example, in the proportion of the population living in low-income households. Data from 2006/07 to 2008/09 showed that one in six people in rural districts live in low-income households, compared to one in four in urban districts. These relatively small differences conceal some systematic dissimilarities. For example, a high proportion of poor people in rural areas are in low-paid jobs. A half of children in urban low-income households have a parent in work, compared with two thirds of children in rural low-income households.

[4] Palmer G (2009) Indicators of poverty and social exclusion in rural England 2009: A report for the Commission for Rural Communities. The Poverty Site. www.poverty.org.uk *retrieved 5 September 2012.*

In rural areas there is a difference in the prevalence of mental health problems amongst wealthier and poor people. Poor people have worse mental health, as is the case in cities. However, the difference between the high- and low-income groups is smaller in rural than in urban populations. Overall, living in a rural area is associated with better mental health than living in an urban environment.

'Common mental disorders' is a term for conditions associated with mild to moderate anxiety and depression that generally can be treated within primary care. The rural population is at lower risk of reporting common mental disorders (Riva *et al.*, 2010). This is particularly true of those in employment. The effect of employment in rural areas in reducing the risk of these disorders is greater than it is in urban areas.

Schizophrenia is less common in rural districts, irrespective of income. A recent study in a rural area of England derived incidence figures for psychosis from referrals to an early intervention service (Kirkbride *et al.*, 2012b). This suggested that not only was the incidence of psychosis lower than in inner-city urban areas, but also that the additional risk arising from minority ethnicity was less pronounced in rural than in urban areas.

Despite the lower prevalence of nearly all mental health problems in rural areas (Nicholson, 2008), suicide is commoner in rural than urban environments. This is especially true in remote and inaccessible areas (Levin & Leyland, 2005). Suicide, however, is not invariably, or even necessarily primarily, associated with mental illness. Suicide rates are known to be strongly affected by social factors, especially unemployment (Yur'yev *et al.*, 2012). This has a much larger effect than poverty alone. Higher rates of suicide amongst the unemployed do not appear to be due to a relationship between mental illness and employment status (Blakely *et al.*, 2003). It is likely that unemployment has a causal role in suicide. However, unemployment is unlikely to be the social factor that accounts for differences in rural and urban suicide rates.

Rural populations are affected by severe stressors of particular types that have little or no impact on people in urban areas. For example, the foot and mouth disease epidemic amongst livestock in 2001 had a catastrophic effect in rural communities but was more or less unnoticeable to urban communities (Peck, 2005).

The existing evidence strongly suggests that whilst poverty and inequality always have a negative effect on well-being, it is not as bad for mental or physical health to grow up in rural poverty as in urban poverty. Some problems are common to poor people living in both environments. Lack of access to transportation may be worse in rural areas, and the costs of transport impose a special financial burden on the rural poor.

There are some evident differences between rural and urban environments that may have importance. Low-cost and social housing in rural areas tends to be located in small enclaves, alongside better quality housing stock. There is no rural equivalent of the large municipal housing estate. As mentioned in Chapter 1 the smallest geographical unit used to analyse routinely collected statistics is the electoral ward. This bundles together very poor and somewhat wealthier areas, obscuring differences between them. This is true in both rural areas and cities. However, it may have a larger effect in masking the impact of poverty in rural areas, as the poor communities involved represent a much smaller proportion of the local population. As a consequence, urban–rural differences may be in part artefacts of comparing large urban areas that are relatively socially homogeneous with smaller rural areas that are more heterogeneous. On the other hand, the impact of poverty may be less severe in rural areas owing to a lower degree of social segregation.

Rural areas have seen a loss of local infrastructure in the same way that poor urban areas have. Village pubs have closed in large numbers, and post office provision has been rationalised and thinned out. It is known that people in the countryside are more positive about the social environment they live in (e.g. McCulloch, 2012). People in rural poverty are not exposed to an unremittingly impoverished or deteriorated environment. They have access to open space and a more attractive physical geography. Rural populations have little choice but to share schools and shops. Access to socially mixed activities is better in small towns and villages. Places of worship, for example, are likely to have congregations from a wide range of occupations and income levels. A critical mass of social disorder is unlikely to arise in small enclaves, which means that exposure to violence and fears about personal safety are less. Gang wars and riots tend not to happen in small towns or the countryside.

Seen in another way, the rural poor, though disadvantaged, may not be exposed to a deteriorated social fabric in the same way as the inner-city poor, and they may be less vulnerable to alienation from mainstream society. It is impossible to say whether these factors are important, but they may be.

Main points in this chapter

1. In developed capitalist nations, the adverse effects of poverty are more closely related to income inequality than to absolute poverty.
2. Although poverty is complex and hard to define, it has consistent and tangible effects on a wide range of health and social problems.
3. Social class remains a valid construct in understanding inequalities.
4. Poverty is not a unitary phenomenon. Urban and rural poverty involve different lifestyles and different problems.

Constellations of disadvantage

Toxteth is an inner-city area just outside of the centre of Liverpool. The housing was constructed in the nineteenth century, a combination of grand homes built for wealthy Victorian merchants and back-to-back working-class terraces built for seafarers, dockers and workers who processed goods as they arrived at the port. The merchants are long gone and port employment more or less disappeared with containerisation in the 1960s. It is one of the most deprived urban areas in the UK, and it has been for some decades. The population is made up of a variety of different groups: a very long-standing Black British community, a similarly well-established Chinese community, and a White population with strong links to Ireland, together with more recently arrived Somali refugees and university students. The rate of male unemployment is extremely high.

The area is both deteriorated and vibrant. Depopulation has left properties 'tinned up' and derelict. There are few shops. Some of the pubs resemble the bar in *Star Wars*. The churches and mosques are well supported. There are numerous community projects. On the other side of Upper Parliament Street, there is magnificent and well-preserved Georgian architecture that is much featured in films and television series.

For mental health professionals working in the area, there is a tangible qualitative difference between Toxteth and adjacent, less-deprived, parts of the city. Some of this difference is a reflection of the effort the population has to make to get by every day. Deprivation is evident, but so is community spirit. The challenge of living in such areas is not about coping with a variety of discrete and independent problems. Instead there is a constellation of disadvantage, whereby problems are inter-related in a complex way. Problems come in bundles. Multiple problems interact with each other and have a combined effect on individual well-being that is greater than the sum of the parts.

One really difficult aspect of inner-city life, and an important component in the resultant constellation of disadvantage, is living with crime. Wilkinson and Pickett (2009) have shown an association between social inequality and crime rates. Criminality leading to conviction is strongly concentrated in the lowest socio-economic classes (SECs). Major organised criminals, wealthy fraudsters and tax evaders reap rewards far in excess of the totality of the returns of everyday crime, but they represent a tiny proportion of all criminal convictions. There appears to be a close link between criminality and perceived economic necessity. If the necessities of life are inaccessible by honest endeavour, it is hardly surprising that some people show little compunction in turning to crime. In any case, alienation from authority weakens social prohibitions. Criminal conviction, shed of its social opprobrium, becomes an occupational hazard to be endured rather than a deterrent. However, crime is perpetrated upon neighbours. Burglaries and car thefts are highest in areas where thieves reside, which tend to be the inner cities. The impact of crime on the fabric of life is multi-faceted.

Aspirations are also affected by constellations of disadvantage, but not necessarily in the form of a poverty of aspiration, as is sometimes suggested by politicians. Wilkinson and Pickett, citing a UNICEF report[1] describe a paradox with regard to childhood ambitions in different countries. When asked about their occupational aspirations, children in more equal societies tend to express lower, more achievable ambitions than children from unequal societies, who express higher and less realisable goals. This may be because smaller income differentials between jobs lead to smaller differences in social status. Practicalities rather than social status may then be more relevant to aspirations. Equally, where it is less possible to gradually move out of poverty, it is understandable that people might pin their hopes on doing so in one mighty bound. The National Lottery, professional football and pop stardom are legal methods of achieving this, and there are prominent role models who have done so. However, very few people can actually find social improvement through these routes.

Crimes such as drug dealing offer a highly profitable business opportunity, and one that is unusual in that it is a particularly accessible activity for people from poor neighbourhoods. However, drug dealing is a dangerous business. Drug dealers have to live with high levels of anxiety. This is a business culture where differences are settled by reference to, or through the use of, firearms. The promise of potential profits is offset by the risk of early death or lengthy imprisonment. Drug dealing and shootings have an awful effect on the wider community. They make everyone feel unsafe and violence tends to escalate. Legitimate businesses, and people who have enough money to choose where to live, shun areas where shootings happen, which further deepens the impoverishment of the area.

There are many other intertwined factors that contribute to the constellations of disadvantage in the inner cities. It is important to recognise that inner cities are not made up of uniformly violent, unruly, self-loathing mobs. On the contrary, our experience of living and working in Toxteth is that the majority of the population are decent, community-minded people who help each other whenever they can and who continue to make attempts to improve the fabric of their neighbourhoods. However, the presence of a critical mass of others whose lifestyles are chaotic

[1] http://www.unicef-irc.org/publications/445 *retrieved 28 May 2013.*

has a strong impact on the quality of life of the whole inner-city population. Drunks, drug addicts and criminals are not an anonymous threat to the decent majority. They are their children, siblings, acquaintances and neighbours. It is easy to imagine that somewhere in this depressing tangle of social adversity there arises a toxic environment that has a permanent effect on people's lives and mental health.

Education

It is an item of faith that the primary legitimate route for people to escape from poverty is education. Selective state-funded grammar schools are nostalgically mourned as the crucible of self-improvement in the post-war period. It is arguable that the peculiarities of the enduring British class system owe their existence to the presence of an undefeated monarchy and attendant aristocracy, which creates a hereditary tier at the top of British society that can only be entered by outsiders with difficulty. Kate Middleton, the Duchess of Cambridge, was an untitled 'commoner', whose marriage into the royal family aroused much comment. Beneath the monarchy there is a fine-grained layering of social groups. Their distinctive characteristics are preserved mainly through the schooling system.

Although the British state educational system started to eliminate selection from the 1960s, the process was never completed. Even in those areas where comprehensive schools offer state education to the full ability range, social mixing has been systematically circumvented. Schools and parents have proved highly creative in ensuring that children do not have to be educated alongside the offspring of the next social class down. This has been achieved by an increase in geographical segregation of social classes, itself partly a consequence of the increased monetary value of residential properties located in the catchment areas of state schools with a good reputation.

Equally important is a private education system that has developed over the past 30 years, catering for a middle-class population that has never made use of the older 'public' school system. We should explain at this point that 'public school' refers to the elite top 10% amongst UK fee-paying schools. Within this group there is a super-elite of nine 'Clarendon Schools' such as Eton College. The peculiar terminology 'public school' arose because these institutions were founded at a time when education was controlled by religious bodies. The new public schools were open to anyone who could pay the fees. They were therefore 'public schools' as opposed to 'ecclesiastical schools'.

British schools reinforce a range of attitudes, aspirations, accent of speech and dialect that may have a more powerful effect on pupils' life prospects than their actual educational attainment, though there is a link between the two. Writing just before the Second World War, George Orwell described himself as 'lower upper middle class' (Orwell, 2001). He was not making a joke. British society has myriad cultural sub-classes, and membership of them has an effect on people's lives and lifestyles.

A third of school leavers go to university, yet social stratification has increased. Not only do different strata have separate schools, they also have separate universities. Until the 1980s, most universities took students from a similar range of class background, with the notable exception of the elite Oxford and Cambridge colleges. The majority of students had attended state grammar schools or public schools. In contrast, there is now intense competition between universities. The perceived value of degrees from different universities varies considerably. This is despite similar curricula and standardised criteria for degree classification. The relabelling of former polytechnics as universities was accompanied by anti-elitist rhetoric, but the effect has, if anything, been in the opposite direction. A steep hierarchy of esteem amongst higher education institutions has emerged. Not only are league tables and consumer guides published, but the 'top' universities aggregate into academic cartels such as the Russell Group. We now have schools for SEC II feeding universities for SEC II. An individual's journey through the educational system is likely to occur mainly in the company of people from a similar background. Taken together with the evidence that social mobility has become far less prevalent than it was in the post-war period, the result is that British society appears to be crystallising into a series of closed, internally homogeneous, strata.

To give just a little of the evidence in support of these assertions from the report of the National Equality Panel (Hills, 2010), those completing higher education at Russell Group universities show marked differences from the demographic profile of students completing higher educations at all UK universities. A significantly higher proportion of men than women go to Russell Group universities. Fifty per cent of private school pupils in higher education go to Russell Group institutions compared with 25% of state school pupils. Amongst students with parents in professional occupations, 40% go to Russell Group institutions, compared with 25% amongst those whose parents hold semi-skilled or unskilled manual jobs. UK-born students of Black, Pakistani and Bangladeshi ethnicity are least likely to go to Russell Group universities.

The earnings of graduates continue to be affected by the same demographic factors that influence which university they attend. After four years in employment, 22% of all male graduates are earning more than £30,000/year; the proportion of female graduates is 12%. Amongst graduates with a private education the proportion is 33% compared with 14% amongst the state educated. Social stratification persists throughout the educational process and on into employment.

Disadvantage generates further disadvantage

The report of the National Equality Panel (Hills, 2010) sets out strong evidence that differences in attainment are rooted in social factors rather than intrinsic ability, which tends to refute the suggestion that class stratification is meritocratic or genetic in origin. In state schools, educational attainment is strongly affected by gender, and females consistently achieve better than males. Ethnicity predicts attainment, but in a complicated way. For example, amongst children who perform at 16 at the national median level of attainment, ethnic minority children are more likely to go on to higher education than white children, but amongst those with high levels of attainment, there is no difference.

Children from backgrounds with low socio-economic status show the highest rates of perinatal factors that adversely affect development, such as low birth weight and maternal post-natal depression, as well as the highest rates of factors within the home that adversely affect development, such as not being read to every day and having no regular bedtime aged three years. At 22 months, children from high socio-economic backgrounds show higher average ability than children from low socio-economic backgrounds. The effect of early developmental disadvantage is amplified as children grow older. By age 10, children with high socio-economic status but low initial ability have overtaken the performance of initial higher ability children from low socio-economic status backgrounds. Participation in higher education, not surprisingly, is closely linked to attainment at 16 years. Children who receive free school meals, but who have high attainment at 16, are less likely than other children to go onto higher education. This reflects a pattern of cumulative and enduring disadvantage as a consequence of growing up in the poorest households that is well established across many domains of everyday life.

The National Equality Panel report showed that children growing up in the inner cities are educationally disadvantaged in a number of different ways. Their parents are unlikely to have been well educated. Children growing up in poverty are less likely than other children to live in households where books are available and where reading is valued as an activity. This is known to create a risk of delayed attainment of literacy skills and may lead on to adult literacy problems. All other educational attainment is highly dependent on literacy.

No matter how well schools perform, they are bound to struggle to lift the attainment of children who are recurrently tested in a system of assessment designed to meet the needs of children from comfortable middle-class homes. Inner-city schools tend to have pupil populations with a peer group culture that is dismissive of educational attainment, which is linked to growing up in an academic monoculture due to stratified schooling. The system of inspection of schools and evaluation of their performance is not especially supportive of schools serving deprived populations. These conditions militate against success for poorer children in the educational system.

Within living memory it was possible to get by in the work place without good literacy skills, or even without any ability to read or write at all. Things have changed. Employment is increasingly dependent on formal educational attainment. In the age of email and the internet, business is increasingly conducted through the written rather than the spoken word. Poor literacy makes life very difficult and the acquisition of knowledge almost impossible. Health education and information is hard to access and retain without literacy. The impact of poor education is exacerbated by misleading ideas and inaccurate information derived from the popular media. Combined with unhealthy lifestyles and high degrees of social stress, the impact of a limited knowledge base is that the poorest are the unhealthiest group in society, with high rates of perinatal mortality, heart disease, lung cancer and, of course, mental illness (Marmot, 2005).

The emergence of 'the underclass'

Over the past 30 years, the problems of the residents of deprived inner cities have markedly worsened against the background of increases in social stratification and other changes to British social structures. This population has always tended to find work in unskilled occupations. The demand for unskilled manual labour has sharply declined. Retail and service industries have increasingly employed unskilled workers on a part-time or casual basis. The combined effects of increasing poverty, educational stratification and a shrinking job market have created major barriers to self-improvement. The rhetoric of the *underclass*, stereotyping the poor as intrinsically unreliable or criminal compounds this. Within inner-city areas a significant part of the population permanently survives outside of paid employment, though they do not always appear in unemployment statistics. There is a distinction in official statistics between the unemployed, the economically active and the economically inactive. Governments have periodically introduced policies that have reduced unemployment figures by moving significant numbers of people into economically inactive categories such as 'invalidity', only to enthusiastically embrace media representations of 'benefit scroungers' when it has been politically expedient to do so.

When vacancies exist in the job market, continued non-employment of a proportion of the population is often cited as evidence that indolence is a cause of unemployment. However, new jobs often require skills and qualifications that the urban working-class population lacks, and in any case new jobs tend to be inaccessible from the inner cities, for example, located far away in peripheral industrial estates, or in distant parts of the UK. Transport and relocation are two modern necessities that are beyond the financial resources of poor people in the inner cities and rural locations alike.

The notion of an *underclass* can be understood in a number of ways. At one end of the political spectrum it is suggested that the benefit system removes all motivation to self-improvement because people are protected from absolute destitution. This traps some people in unproductive dependency. At the other end of the political spectrum, the *underclass* is seen as a rebranding of the victims of an aggressively inequitable and unjust socio-economic system that pushes some people under. If we assume for a moment that the *underclass* represents a valid social group, there is a tension between the two main ways of understanding their disempowerment. To the right, they are disadvantaged by an adverse moral environment characterised by perverse incentives against earning an honest living.

To the left, they are disadvantaged by an adverse social environment characterised by systematic discrimination and exclusion.

To us, the rhetoric of an *underclass* appears to be rooted in a profound antagonism to poor people and a conviction that they are the authors of their own misfortunes. There is strong evidence that the situation of people in lower social classes *has* worsened, and much of the evidence is set out in the report of the National Equality Panel (Hills, 2010). For example, comparisons made in 1946, 1958, 1970 and 2000 showed a progressive change in the social position of women living in social housing. In 1946, they were much more likely to be working mothers than women living in owner-occupied homes. By 1970, this had changed and the proportions were equal. In 2000, few women in social housing were working mothers. Living in social housing had become more strongly associated with poverty. Furthermore, over the last 30 years social mobility, measured in terms of personal income compared to parental income, has sharply declined.

The UK has higher rates of social problems associated with poverty than most other European countries. The domestic political agenda is dominated by concerns over lawlessness, drug taking, indolence, and other social ills, which are generally attributed to the disorderly poor. Those in poverty are referred to using unmistakably pejorative labels such as 'chavs' or 'neighbours from hell'. The concern over the effect that the unruly mob has on honest citizens has been so great that in 1998 the Labour government introduced a system of summary justice to control them, known as Anti-Social Behaviour Orders (ASBOs). ASBOs are civil law orders that are applied in response to behaviour that is deemed antisocial though not necessarily criminal. ASBOs impose restrictions on the behaviour of the individual. Breach of these restrictions is a criminal offence, punishable by up to five years imprisonment. At the time of writing ASBOs are being reviewed with the suggestion that they are replaced by a Criminal Behaviour Order and a Crime Prevention Injunction.

As the social structure of Britain has altered in recent decades, attitudes to the most deprived part of the population have also changed. Broadly speaking, for most of the twentieth century, people living in deprivation were regarded as people *with* problems. More recently they have come to be seen as people who *are* a problem. Where interventions were once based on philanthropy, charity or social action, they are now increasingly coercive and punitive. In parallel, there has been a substantial increase in the prison population (according to government figures, almost doubling from 44,975 in 1990 to 85,951 in 2011).[2] In the 1960s there was a television play called 'Cathy Come Home' which was concerned with a family that becomes homeless and is forcibly split up. At the time the response was an outcry over the plight of homeless people, which led to the formation of a large charity, Shelter, to assist them. By the 1990s homelessness was commonly portrayed as being associated with undesirable behaviours, such as aggressive

---

[2] Berman G (2012) *Prison population statistics*. Standard Note SN/SG/4334. London: House of Commons Library. www.parliament.uk/briefing-papers/SN04334.pdf *retrieved 28 May 2013*.

begging and drug addiction. This shift is evident in attitudes to a wide group of people struggling with major social problems.

The mainstream political consensus is that poverty and its associated problems are not due to social policies or the economic depression, but a consequence of bad choices and undesirable personal characteristics of the poor. These include benefit dependency, bad parenting and a criminal sub-culture. Their moral deficiencies are claimed to be a major cause of a budget deficit that just happened to become problematic after billions of pounds were used to bail out failing banks. Owen Jones has written a passionate book analysing the change in attitudes to the poor (Jones, 2012). He suggests that the spread of the use of the word 'chav', a pejorative term for working-class people, their tastes and their behaviours, is emblematic of a general demonisation of the working class. Jones sees this as part of a progressive assault that commenced with the neutralisation of trade unions by the Thatcher government.

Jones characterises the process as a successful class war waged by the political representatives of the property-owning class. According to this view, their confidence in attacking the poorest part of the population increased when the fall of communism removed the threat that civil discontent could lead to the spread of anti-capitalist regimes. The threat of revolution may seem implausible now, but in the late 1960s and early 1970s revolutionary movements were aggressively suppressed in countries as different as Chile and France. According to Jones, low-wage economics, cultural demonisation and growing inequality are intrinsic elements of a political monoculture that views increasing wealth for the few as a legitimate political objective.

The *underclass* concept represents the re-emergence of an ancient tradition of despising the poorest. It has a close correspondence to the Lumpenproletariat as described by Karl Marx. He was invariably rude and dismissive about this group at the bottom of society. The currency of the *underclass* concept implicitly suggests a return to the ideas of Social Darwinism. This is a doctrine (or more correctly, a set of related doctrines) that originated in Europe. It was influential amongst intellectuals in the first half of the twentieth century. It was closely linked to eugenics, with prominent adherents on both the right and the left of the political spectrum. After the Second World War, Nazi crimes made discussion of Social Darwinism and eugenics unacceptable. These terms took on a sinister connotation.

The central proposition of Social Darwinism is that social survival of the fittest leads to the most able being at the top of society and the least able at the bottom. On the assumption that ability is determined by genetic factors, 'good' genes aggregate in higher social classes and 'bad' genes in lower classes. Following this logic, the problems of those at the bottom of society are due to an accumulation of genetic inferiority. The great concern of those who adhered to these ideas was that modern man was no longer exposed to evolutionary pressure. Far from being bred out of the population, bad genes were proliferating and undermining the national genetic stock, because poor people had more children than wealthy people. Even twentieth-century progressives with impeccable credentials as champions of social justice, such as George Bernard Shaw and Marie Stopes, had worries about this.

Social Darwinism is based on bad genetics. The assumption that human ability and behaviour is rigidly determined by genetic legacy is far from established, or even necessarily credible, despite strong support for socio-biology from some prominent geneticists such as Richard Dawkins. Even those human characteristics that are predominantly genetically determined, such as height, are polygenic. As such they are subject to regression to the mean. Parents whose place in the ability spectrum is far from the mean produce offspring who are, in general, closer to the population average than their parents were. The assumption that social position is determined by ability can be convincingly refuted by reference to the British royal family.

Another atavistic but intrinsic element to the *underclass* concept is moral decline. Politicians and others have recurrently attributed the social ills that affect poor people to a breakdown in adherence to moral values and codes of behaviour. This is seen in the breakdown of traditional family structures, in a loss of adherence to religious faith and in a 'nanny' welfare state that cushions the wayward from the consequences of their actions (i.e. destitution). In the British general election of 2010, the Conservative party claimed that Britain was a 'broken society' as a consequence of moral turpitude.

There is little evidence that new family structures are damaging or cause chaos, social disorder or social problems. For example, Scandinavia has enthusiastically embraced new patterns of family life whilst avoiding British levels of social problems.[3] Similarly, the nanny state argument is unsustainable in the face of the evidence that the most equal nations, with the most generous welfare provision, have some of the lowest rates of social problems in the developed world.

Restoration of traditional or religious values is a theme in this 'moral decline' school of thought.[4] The argument that religion and spirituality are necessary to human happiness has become so pervasive that psychiatric journals now regularly publish papers advocating that spirituality or religion should be integrated with psychiatric practice as a necessary and essential component (Poole & Higgo, 2011). Whilst it is undeniable that religion provides comfort, meaning and social structure for millions, there is also good evidence that it causes a good deal of social harm, for example, through sectarian conflict. It is particularly difficult to believe that Anglicanism could offer solutions to social problems at a time when it appears to be ripping itself apart over controversies concerning homosexuality and women priests.

---

[3] Ventura S (2009) *Changing patterns of nonmarital childbearing in the United States.* NCHS Data Brief No 18 US National Center for Health Statistics www.cdc.gov/nchs/data/databriefs/db18.pdf *retrieved 28 May 2013.*

[4] Carey G (2011) *Staying grounded in a world of shaking foundations.* Speech, St Martin's Episcopal Church, Houston, USA. www.glcarey.co.uk/speeches/2011/houston3.html *retrieved 6 September 2012.*

The *underclass* is alleged to take lots of drugs and to drink too much (see Chapter 6). Heavy drinking is not particularly common in the lowest social classes. In fact per capita alcohol consumption is greater in higher social classes than lower ones (Office of National Statistics, 2006). Epidemics of substance misuse have repeatedly been held to be the cause of the social problems of the poor. In the eighteenth century there was a panic that cheap gin was causing widespread social problems by destroying the moral behaviour of the working-class population. Similar ideas drove the temperance movement, which was successful in banning alcohol in the USA during the 1920s, the so-called 'Prohibition era'. Whilst Prohibition did reduce per capita alcohol consumption in the USA, it proved disastrously counter-productive through placing the production and distribution of alcohol in the hands of organised crime.

For many years there has been concern over drug use, believed by many policy makers to be responsible for social ills from crime to schizophrenia. Whilst drug addiction is not a good thing either for individuals or for society in general, there is little evidence that it is a primary cause of the problems of the urban poor. Put another way, if all access to illegal drugs could be abolished, there would be benefits for some individuals, but the generality of the social difficulties of poor people would be substantially unchanged. To take two bits of evidence in support of this, there is good reason to suppose that the extent to which crime is conducted primarily in order to fund drug habits is routinely overestimated (Stevens, 2008). Figures extrapolated from the most criminal section of the drug-taking population are bound to be misleading, as they fail to take sufficient account of the fact that many drug users do not pay for drugs through crime.

There is an assumption that if people did not take drugs, they would not be criminals. However, the risk factors for drug addiction and criminality are similar to each other. For many people, criminality and drug taking are not in a causal relationship (Stevens, 2007). Instead, they have similar origins. People who have an inability to make and follow plans tend to be attracted to rapid and easy rewards without reference to later consequences. Drug use and crime are, in this respect, similar to each other. We explore the relationship between cannabis use and schizophrenia in Chapter 5.

Migration

Migration remains a contentious and fiercely debated political issue in the UK, although railing against migration is as meaningful as objecting to the existence of money; it is possible to imagine a world without migration or without money, but neither is at all likely to happen. Relatively free movement of people is an intrinsic feature of the world economy. Scapegoating migrants for social problems is a deeply ingrained and disreputable bad habit that British politicians condemn in others, but freely indulge in themselves when it is expedient to do so. Migration has always been a feature of city life. Indeed, cities were formed by migrants in the first place. If migration has increased in pace, this is mainly a reflection of globalisation. The free movement of commodities and labour is a pre-requisite for capitalism to grow, and if capitalism does not grow, it shrinks, with catastrophic economic consequences.

As wealthier workers have moved away from the inner cities they have been replaced by newly arrived migrants, who tend to settle close to each other. Multi-culturalism is a prominent feature of inner-city life. In many areas it generates a vibrancy that offsets some of the grim deterioration of the inner city. Migrants, and more particularly their children, undergo a mutual assimilation with estab-lished inner-city populations. There are reciprocal benefits for these communities in terms of access to cultural traditions, kinship networks and social support resources. However, a significant sub-group that regards itself as the indigenous population bitterly resents the presence of migrants and attributes the problems of their neighbourhoods to immigration. Some of this resentment is due to racism, white supremacist beliefs or tension between different minority ethnic communi-ties. Much of it is xenophobic with fear of difference and change. This creates a constituency for neo-fascists, who feed on these attitudes to create the appearance of being the only political force that is sympathetic to the special problems of a neglected 'white working class'.

Migrants tend to exist outside of clear class structures, at least for the first generation. As we have seen, migration has health consequences for the offspring of some groups of migrants, which are additional to other socio-economic dis-advantage (see Chapter 2). One possible explanation for this is that growing up alongside a threatening and aggressively racist sub-population, combined with experience of more subtle but pervasive institutional racism, creates its own spe-cific type of social adversity. As mentioned in Chapter 1, the effect of ethnicity as a risk factor for schizophrenia is ameliorated by living amongst larger num-bers of people from the same ethnic background (Kirkbride *et al.*, 2007). This would tend to support the view that the special factor is exposure to racism and discrimination.

Homelessness

Homelessness is an extreme example of a constellation of disadvantage. Studies of the homeless population has shown reasonably consistent findings in modern times.[5] Single homeless people are predominantly young males. People from ethnic minorities were once under-represented, but are now over-represented. Although the proportion of women is small, it is growing. The group of older people who conform to a traditional stereotype of vagrancy, 'tramps' or 'bag ladies', is small. The single homeless population has high rates of alcohol and drug dependency

[5] Palmer G (2012) The Poverty Site: Homelessness. http://www.poverty.org.uk/81/index.shtml
retrieved 1 October 2012.

(about 70%) and of mental illness (between 30 and 70%). Many individuals have both an addiction and a mental illness. There is a small population of people who are homeless solely because of symptoms of mental illness. For most homeless people, mental illness is one of a number of severe problems in their life. It is not necessarily their worst problem (Harding *et al.*, 2011; Poole & Fleming, 2005).

People continue to sleep rough in the UK, but homelessness is not the same as rooflessness.[6] For the most part homelessness is a matter of very unstable housing. Episodes of rough sleeping tend to be brief but recurrent. Individuals move between homelessness hostels, rough bed and breakfast establishments, prison, the street and friends' sofas. The two key factors that maintain this pattern of homelessness are persistent behaviours that others find hard to tolerate and a difficulty in adjusting to a settled lifestyle. Health and social care services for the homeless have to be exceptionally flexible and creative in the way that they work. It is difficult to resolve homeless people's problems to the point where they can resettle in permanent accommodation.

Homeless people are very likely to have had abusive or difficult childhoods, and many have been in local authority care (Harding *et al.*, 2011). Their education has often been disrupted by recurrent changes of school or by exclusion because of early difficult behaviour. Their educational attainment tends to be poor or non-existent. Many raise money through begging, shop-lifting or sex work. This brings them into conflict with the law, and they are over-represented in the prison population. Not only are they perpetrators of crime, they are also victims of crime. In particular they are frequent victims of violent crime. A significant minority are ex-service personnel.

Homeless people have difficulty in sustaining relationships, which tend to be brief, intense and volatile. Where there is substance misuse, this is frequently chaotic and involves combinations of substances, most prominently heroin, cocaine and alcohol. They survive on bad diets and they are often heavy smokers. They have poor physical health and a high mortality rate. This is roughly six times higher than the general population, including from violence, accidental overdose and suicide (Nielsen *et al.*, 2011). Many show evidence of personality disorder, although the environment that they live in is so abnormal that it can be hard to assess personality in isolation from their other problems.

Not all homeless people have all of these problems, but most have several of them. Causality is complex. For example, some become substance-dependent as a consequence of mixing with a large number of substance misusers in the homeless population. They steal to buy alcohol, get arrested and go to prison where drugs can be easier to obtain than alcohol. The various difficulties interact with each other. Even when someone is successfully resettled they retain links with other

---

[6] Homeless Link (2012) Homeless Facts and Figures. http://homeless.org.uk/facts *retrieved 1 October 2012.*

homeless people, who will often use the new accommodation for purposes that are in conflict with tenancy agreements. Allowing friends who are noisy unruly drug users to share accommodation can easily lead to eviction and a return to homelessness.

Living on the margins of society is an existence where daily survival is the dominant concern. Most of the settled population take it for granted that it is sensible to plan for the future, to take action to protect their health and to follow long-term objectives through stepwise strategies. To a homeless person, worrying about the future lacks salience in the face of the pressing need to get by each day. Patterns of recurrently making short-sighted bad decisions look feckless and unintelligent to a middle-class health professional. However, a homeless person is likely to see long- and medium-term goals as unattainable. A decision to spend money on alcohol to be shared with friends rather than saving it for a rent deposit on a flat is not as irrational as it may at first appear. Long experience of failure may suggest to them that they are likely to remain homeless for the foreseeable future, and that their largesse regarding alcohol is likely to be reciprocated when others have money and they do not.

Homeless people are a small proportion of the population and they are at the bottom of society. It is not surprising that they suffer from a high rate of severe difficulties. Constellations of disadvantage also affect less severely deprived populations, including people living in urban deprivation. These constellations cause difficulties, sustain them and obstruct their resolution.

High-risk populations

There have been recent efforts to identify smaller and more specific groups in the population ('social segments') who are at high risk of various types of problems, largely as a consequence of the growing interest in 'social marketing'. One part of social marketing is based upon the seemingly self-evident concept that public health interventions are most efficiently targeted at high-risk groups, where modification of undesirable behaviour or lifestyles might lead to substantial reductions in rates of social and health problems in the general population.

Social segments can be identified through a range of routinely collected data sources, such as the National Census, Office for National Statistics data and commercial intelligence on consumption. Although social marketing has a common-sense appeal, as it allows interventions to be directed to those parts of the population most in need of them, almost all studies evaluating such an approach are quasi-experimental (i.e. they lack a control group). Whilst there is evidence that the approach may work in some public health programmes (Lowry et al., 2009), this does not necessarily imply that it is the most appropriate approach under all circumstances. For some problems there is a very small population at high risk and a big population at low or medium risk. The largest numbers of cases arise in the latter group, whose behaviour is modified more easily than those who are at highest risk. Strategies aimed at the highest-risk group may not have the greatest preventative impact. For example, suicide prevention strategies that apply to the whole population appear to be more effective than campaigns targeted at specific high-risk groups (Pitman & Caine, 2012). Reasons for this include the presence of a far larger number of people at medium risk than at high risk; difficulty in identifying those at high risk; and a greater resistance to intervention amongst high-risk individuals.

Social marketing approaches cause discomfort to those who believe that the solutions to socially determined problems should be found by changing social structures. Targeted health information as a method of inducing healthier behaviours or lifestyle choices seems to imply a model of understanding public health as a matter of aggregated individual decisions. Social marketing is attractive to governments with a strong attachment to the market as a solution to economic and social problems. After several decades of social marketing, there is no real evidence that it can produce more than piecemeal change in widespread socially determined problems. Social marketing is bound to struggle to alter problems related to constellations of disadvantage, where multiple problems play against each other.

Sophisticated data bases on social segmentation have developed as a consequence of the commercial use of information technology. Data generated by the use of credit, debit and loyalty cards allows companies to collect information about patterns of consumption, and to link market segments (i.e. households with specific consumer patterns) with post codes. This provides companies with information about the demography and likely lifestyle of households grouped together into very small geographical areas, which allows very precise targeting of marketing effort.

Such data bases generate fine-grain typologies of demography, income and lifestyle, and can link these to neighbourhood-level geography. In addition to their intended function in marketing, it is evident that these commercial resources could be exploited to understand health inequalities (Morleo *et al.*, 2010b). This creates interesting possibilities, though the use of commercial data bases is problematic. On the one hand, the lack of an underlying theory makes this approach scientifically attractive, as the groupings are generated by data on consumption patterns, not on preconceptions as to how and why lifestyles form into categories. On the other hand, there are groups of people who do not appear on these data bases, such as those poor people who exclusively deal in cash, and the very rich who do not use the same retail and banking infrastructure as the rest of the population. This is not a problem to the companies which have established the data bases, as neither group is likely to be accessible or influenced by mainstream marketing. It is a much bigger problem in using the data to study health inequalities or to target populations at very high risk of mental health problems, as they are one of the major groups who don't use credit cards, loyalty cards or, in many cases, bank accounts.

The interface between models of poverty and policy formation

Political understandings of poverty are strongly influenced by moral judgements and the application of values. It appears to be impossible for politicians to address poverty without taking sides. The right, broadly speaking, take the side of the rich, or as they would prefer it, the wealth generators. Their general response to the poor is that poverty is a problem that they themselves generate, that it is caused by their own behaviour, and that if they behaved more like the rich, their situation would improve. The left, on the other hand, take the side of the poor, and understand poverty as something that is accidentally or deliberately inflicted on them by the rich. It is of note that no mainstream political party in the UK currently takes the latter position as part of their main policy platform.

It is possible to separate oneself from preconceptions of this sort. The evidence suggests that poverty is not an inevitable or immutable feature of society. It is entirely clear that a high level of income inequality is bad for individuals' health and social well-being, and that this, in turn, is bad for society as a whole. Structural solutions to problems related to poverty appear to be much more effective than piecemeal responses, but they have become profoundly unpopular with mainstream UK politicians. This is presumably because they are seen, almost certainly correctly, as incompatible with optimal national economic performance. It may be reasonable to construe the dilemma thus: are social and health inequalities, which are currently worsening, sufficiently important to justify the sacrifice of any element of national wealth generation?

Main points in this chapter

1. Serious and enduring poverty arises as part of constellations of disadvantage whereby multiple problems interact.
2. The educational system reflects and sustains a high degree of social stratification.
3. Disadvantage generates further disadvantage. Bright children from poor backgrounds progressively underachieve.
4. The concept of the *underclass* reiterates historical patterns of demonising poor people. It is associated with punitive social policies.
5. Migrants and their offspring are additionally disadvantaged through explicit and implicit racism.
6. Homelessness is part of a particularly severe constellation of disadvantage. Homeless people can be difficult to help and tend to die young.

4

Depression and anxiety

There is an international consensus that depression is becoming the leading public health problem of our time, a major cause of disability and impaired productivity in the high-income countries (National Collaborating Centre for Mental Health, 2010), and perhaps an even bigger problem in middle- and low-income countries (Demyttenaere *et al.*, 2004). In the course of a lifetime, almost everyone has some experience of anxiety and depression, albeit at relatively mild levels of intensity for most people. In contrast, the majority of the population have no first-hand experience of the symptoms of non-affective mental illnesses such as schizophrenia. Everyday experience of affective symptoms leads to a common understanding of cause and effect. An intimate relationship between the stresses of life and symptoms of affective disorders seems obvious. Poverty is stressful and common sense would dictate that it tends to be associated with high levels of anxiety and depression.

There is an established association between a range of social factors (most of which have a clear association with poverty) and depression. The work of Wilkinson and Pickett (2009) has shown a general trend towards more depression where there is greater income inequality, although they acknowledge that this relationship is not a perfect fit. There are statistics on the rates of treatment for depression in developed economies that correspond to these findings. Most treatment of anxiety and depression occurs in primary care settings. In a 2007 household survey (Office for National Statistics, 2009) 23% of adults in England reported that they had at least one psychiatric disorder, generally anxiety or depression. Antidepressants are the most commonly prescribed medications in the USA, and rates of antidepressant prescribing have steadily increased in the UK, despite increased availability of non-drug treatments under the Improving Access to Psychological Therapies (IAPT) initiative (NHS Health and Social Care Information Centre, 2012).

Severe anxiety and major depression have the key features of illnesses. They are disproportionate to the circumstances that provoke them; they are self-sustaining; they can lead to death. Lesser degrees of depression and anxiety are part of normal experience. It is far from clear whether everyday anxiety and depression exist on a continuum with the illness syndromes. The experience of anxiety and depression cannot be accepted as necessarily indicative of mental illnesses. Conflating feelings of anxiety and depression with mental illness turns the relationship between social adversity and depression from an association into a tautology. Difficult lives make people unhappy; what else do you expect? There is a strong tendency to rely upon technological solutions to human unhappiness when it is labelled illness. There is a prima facie case that where the origins of unhappiness lie in social conditions, it would be better to address these directly, either at the individual or at the societal level. The illusion of solutions through therapeutic intervention may be damaging.

Depression as an illness

Until the 1960s, psychiatry regarded anxiety and depression as separate conditions. Three main subtypes of depression were recognised. The first was manic-depression, now known as bipolar affective disorder, which is still regarded as a separate disease entity. The second was a severe form of depression that tended to recurrence in the absence of episodes of mania. It was characterised by biological features such as sleep disturbance, and was often associated with mood-congruent delusions. This was variously known as melancholia, psychotic depression or endogenous depression. The term 'endogenous' reflected the belief that the condition lacked external antecedents. Sir Aubrey Lewis gave a lucid historical account of melancholia in a seminal paper (Lewis, 1934). Finally, there was neurotic or reactive depression that was essentially a response to social and psychological circumstances.

The 1960s and 1970s were a period when psychiatric nosology was subject to intense research effort. Although the model of three distinct types of depression corresponded to clinical experience, it was difficult to find supporting evidence for systematic differences between two (or more) distinct types of unipolar depression. Indeed, it was difficult to show that depression and anxiety clustered into separate disorders. The 'endogenous' nature of depression was called into question as evidence accumulated that relapse was associated with antecedent adversity, mainly through life-event research.

Robert Kendell summarised the evidence in the mid 1970s (Kendell, 1976), noting that there was continuing confusion over the nosology of depression. He concluded that whilst researchers had repeatedly suggested that the endogenous syndrome represented a real, separate, diagnostic entity, it was difficult to find evidence for distinct non-endogenous categories of depression. Conditions that appeared to be a response to life circumstances tended to be characterised by a mixture of anxiety and depressive symptoms, and they didn't fall into clear diagnostic syndromes. He suggested that a dimensional model, with operational criteria, was more appropriate than the use of categories of uncertain validity. Since that time there has been a de facto acceptance that the difference between different sub-types of depression is largely one of severity. This has been encouraged by the development of the concept of major depression in the international classification systems, with diagnostic symptom clusters being identified to allow an atheoretical and descriptive classification of other affective disorders.

There can be no doubt that psychiatric nosology and diagnosis lacked rigour prior to the development of operationalised criteria, but modern diagnostic systems are far from ideal. They are intrinsically dependent on symptoms, and neglect the link between mood, personality, social factors and cultural context. It is fair to say that they drain meaning from diagnostic formulation. As they are purely descriptive, someone suffering from a discrete episode of illness can easily meet criteria for two or more disorders, for example, major depression and panic disorder (Maj, 2005). Older ways of thinking about psychiatric diagnosis recognised a hierarchy, whereby more severe disorders could lead to symptoms of less severe disorders. This was a sustainable and logical position. The idea that someone might, as if by coincidence, happen to have two entirely separate axis I disorders simultaneously is plainly nonsensical. The potentially misleading division of one disorder into several symptom cluster diagnoses might be expected to encourage multiple parallel treatments rather than single overarching treatment strategies.

Psychiatry has a continuing problem in understanding less severe forms of depression and distinguishing this from everyday emotional distress. This complicates the task of understanding the relationship between poverty and depression.

A brief overview of criticisms of the concept of mental illness

The validity of the concept of mental illness has long been debated. There are continuing controversies over the distinction between mental illness and mental distress. Psychiatry stands accused of being preoccupied with 'mental illness' and of having little interest in mental well-being.

Anti-psychiatry

Thomas Szasz died in 2012 at the age of 92. He was a man of extraordinary energy and, it must be said, dogmatic certainty. He published and campaigned from the 1950s right up until the time of his death. He insisted that the concept of mental illness is a logical nonsense and that it is scientifically invalid (see, for example Szasz, 2007). To Szasz, a priori illnesses had to have a basis in physiology and pathology. According to Szasz, as the mind is not an organ of the body, it cannot be diseased. Szasz believed that mental illness was merely a legal or social label used by authority, mainly in the form of the state, to marginalise and stigmatise people who do not conform. He drew a parallel between the modern use of psychiatric diagnoses and accusations of witchcraft in the past. He strongly objected to all forms of compulsory treatment and detention for mental illness. He did not accept that there were any grounds to regard people as lacking responsibility for their actions, no matter how irrational or 'ill' they might seem. He was opposed to the use of legal defences against conviction for offences committed when 'mentally ill', including the insanity plea and diminished responsibility (Szasz, 1966). He was a right-wing libertarian, who believed that a legitimate relationship between a doctor and patient, or between therapist and client, should of necessity be commercial. On occasion he worked closely with surprising allies, including the Church of Scientology (Watts, 2012).

Michel Foucault was probably the most famous of the so-called 'post-modernists' (although he rejected the label). He developed a similar, though more diverse, set of ideas from a left-wing viewpoint, based on an interpretation of history that has proven to be highly contentious. To him, whilst ideas about mental illness go back to antiquity, the modern concept was developed during the Enlightenment, when rationalism emerged as the predominant ideology of Capitalism (see for example, Foucault, 2005). According to Foucault, in developed countries the dominant social stratum controls the way society thinks about itself. The ruling elite uses a rationalist ideology to lend the legitimacy of abstracted logic to the (to him false) suggestion that those who refuse to conform (a moral decision) are diseased (a biological malfunction). To Foucault, mental illness is a concept which is intrinsically marginalising, as it invalidates the meaning of individuals' actions. The social function of the mental health system is to nullify non-conformity. The apparently philanthropic motives for the establishment of mental hospitals in the early part of the nineteenth century was actually part of 'the Great Confinement', which allowed the authorities to form psychiatric concentration camps, industrialising the brutalisation of 'deviant' minorities.

Although both Szasz and Foucault have attracted a great deal of attention, neither fares well in the face of the test of empiricism. Szasz's arguments rest on an idiosyncratic definition of disease or illness that demands that the physiology of a condition must be known before it can be regarded as a disease. His refusal to accept 'excuses' for behaviour driven by psychosis is hard to swallow for anyone familiar with the realities of serious mental illness. Foucault's account of the Great Confinement has been condemned as incompatible with known historical fact. Both models depend on a degree of circular reasoning and ignore substantial bodies of evidence. Neither model can cope very well with the undeniable and awkward reality that people labelled as suffering from mental illness rarely behave in ways that threaten the overall social order to any noticeable extent.

R.D. Laing was, broadly speaking, a libertarian of the New Left. His early work, which asserted that the things that people with schizophrenia say are not non-sensical but meaningful, was a sound clinical observation, albeit framed in the language of existential phenomenology (Laing, 1965). It does not seem controversial 50 years later. However, he went on to become the best known of a group of mainly British psychiatrists who regarded psychosis as an understandable response to an irrational social environment. At some points in his career he advocated that psychosis should be embraced and worked through. Laing changed his position quite frequently (for example, towards the end of his life he acknowledged that antipsychotic medication was helpful) and many of the better known aspects of his writing linked with the New Age movement, which, in congruence with the psychedelic preoccupations of the time, was concerned with people's inner life, dream worlds and personal growth (Laing, 1967). These elements of his thinking have not stood the test of time, not least because of the complete absence of evidence for the transformative benefits of suffering from a serious mental illness.

The older critiques of a psychiatric 'medical model' (i.e. those originating in ideas developed in the 1960s and 1970s) have a lot in common with each other. They tend to the view that psychiatry is intrinsically oppressive, not just through brutalising actions (such as involuntary treatment), but through the intrinsic qualities of its underlying concepts. They see mental illness as an accusation rather than as a diagnosis. They rarely accept the value of conventional treatment and tend to see it as inappropriate or abusive. They are concerned about the social marginalisation of people *accused* of being mentally ill. In so far as they offer any solutions for people suffering from mental illness, they advocate an altered relationship between the 'mentally ill' and the rest of society, ranging from treating emotional well-being as a free market commodity through to finding emancipation in the notion that there is nothing wrong with being psychotic. None can rely on replicable evidence to support their claims. They challenge orthodoxy at the level of values, for example, with regard to the validity of concepts of psychopathology or as to whether it is ever right to restrict liberty and autonomy by reason of mental illness. These critiques can be taken to implicitly suggest that the relationship between mental illness and poverty is self-evident and embedded in invalid concepts. Indeed, they suggest that the concept of mental illness is an attempt to invalidate the legitimate discontent of the marginalised or impoverished.

Contemporary challenges to organised psychiatry

Although the antipsychiatry movement of the 1970s proved to be something of a dead end from the practical point of view, as it offered very little tangible comfort or help to people in mental distress, there were some positive developments that had their origins in challenges to psychiatric orthodoxy (for example, therapeutic communities). The tradition of the critique of psychiatry continues unabated, and it continues to have some positive effects. Older movements were mostly led by renegade psychiatrists, who became famous, but whose ideas had little impact on their profession or upon practice in mental health services. There is now a vigorous patient-led consumer movement that has been highly effective in bringing about changes in attitudes in mental health services. It is hard to know the extent to which they have succeeded in getting services to improve, but they have certainly tried very hard. We discuss these service user-led developments in Chapters 8 and 9.

The contemporary manifestations of the dissident professional movement travel under a range of labels and with varying degrees of engagement with the psychiatric mainstream. In the UK a proportion of them sit within the broad umbrella of the Critical Psychiatry Network.[1] The Network share concerns about psychiatric practice where and when it is heavily dependent upon psychiatric classification and the use of pharmaceuticals. They believe that psychiatric diagnosis has poor construct validity and they are sceptical of the value of medication as a treatment modality. They are interested in the study of relationships, meaning and narrative.

None of these concerns are necessarily outside of the psychiatric mainstream, as they are shared by many social psychiatrists. However, the tone of their rhetoric is unmistakably iconoclastic. One can be left with a lingering suspicion that they sometimes tilt at windmills by attacking concepts that lack general currency within the profession (for example, the concept that mental illness is fundamentally due to a chemical imbalance) (Moncrieff, 2006). They distinguish themselves from anti-psychiatrists such as Szasz, by reference to their pragmatism and acknowledgement of suffering. They share with him discomfort over coercion, social control and decontextualisation. The Network includes Pat Bracken and Phil Thomas, who have developed 'post-psychiatry', an attempt to introduce post-modernism to psychiatric practice (Bracken & Thomas, 2009). Philosophically, the Network declares itself to have concerns over the limitations of positivism and phenomenology, and over the waning of hermeneutics.

There are two particular critiques of modern psychiatry that are of special relevance to the relationship between poverty and mental illness. The first is the idea that depression is a modern invention, that it is not so much a mental disorder as a marketing strategy of the pharmaceutical industry. The second is the related but distinct idea that human distress has been increasingly medicalised, and hence decontextualized, in high-income countries.

David Healy is a professor of psychiatry who has long been a prominent critic of the pharmaceutical industry. Returning to debates over the nosology of depression, Healy takes the view that there is a core authentic severe affective disorder that used to be known as melancholia, characterised by depressed mood, biological changes and a tendency to psychotic symptoms, essentially the same syndrome that Kendell called endogenous depression. It tends to respond to physical treatments, such as electroconvulsive therapy. According to Healy, the pharmaceutical industry, having developed antidepressant drugs, has expanded the limits of the diagnosis of depression. They have increased the indications for the use of their products far beyond any supportable boundaries. Initially there was a proliferation in the number of sub-types of depression, and more recently entirely new disease entities have been devised.

Although Healy has published empirical evidence to support his thesis (e.g. Linden et al., 2011; Harris et al., 2011), he is essentially a medical historian and polemicist. He appears to regard the alleged behaviour of the pharmaceutical industry as a mixture of conspiracy and moral failure. There is a problematic temporal gap between the work by Kendell and others that led to a major change in

---

[1] http://www.criticalpsychiatry.co.uk/ *retrieved 29 May 2013.*

the way that depression was conceptualised in the 1970s, and the alleged disease-mongering of Big Pharma in response to the development of selective serotonin reuptake inhibitor (SSRI) antidepressants in the 1980s. This gap creates a problem for the conspiracy theory, which is similar to anachronisms that mar Foucault's reasoning. Flaws in Healy's rhetoric do not invalidate the argument that antidepressants are currently prescribed for many people who cannot benefit from them, as they do not suffer from depression of a type or severity that would indicate a good response.

There is widespread concern within psychiatry over a proliferation of psychiatric diagnoses and a broadening of diagnostic boundaries. For example, some estimates of the prevalence of bipolar affective disorder have been revised upwards from approximately 0.5% of the population to 10% (Smith *et al.*, 2011). There is a game, popular amongst cynical psychiatrists, of adding together the highest estimates of prevalence of attention deficit hyperactivity disorder (ADHD), bipolar affective disorder, Asperger's syndrome, *forme fruste* schizophrenia, borderline personality disorder and so on. The total is well in excess of 100% which suggests that not only is good mental health an unrealisable dream, one should be grateful for meeting the criteria for just one disorder, as most people suffer from several. Notwithstanding the mischievous intention of this exercise, there are real problems in suggesting that a substantial proportion of the entire population are mentally unwell, not least because it suggests, on the one hand, that intervention might be appropriate for a very large number of people or, on the other hand, that mental disorder is an intrinsic aspect of the human condition that just has to be endured.

Derek Summerfield is a psychiatrist with first-hand experience of work with people and populations affected by war, atrocity and torture (Summerfield, 2000). He has been highly critical of the medicalisation of distress, and of what he regards as systematic exaggerations of the level of the global burden of mental illness. Whilst many other commentators have focussed on the role of the pharmaceutical industry, Summerfield has been equally critical of the indiscriminate use of psychological therapies and other interventions that, in his view, undermine the resilience of communities and their ability to cope with trauma through their own resources. He has criticised the construct validity of post-traumatic stress disorder, suggesting that it was devised to meet the needs of the US legal system when it faced compensation claims following the Vietnam War (Summerfield, 2001). Summerfield's central point is that medicalising distress, and seeking to intervene to alter reactions that are intrinsically self-limiting, is damaging to communities. Medicalisation fosters the idea that all distress requires a professional intervention and thus creates disability. Significant parts of a population subject to trauma find themselves very distressed. Akin to grief, they might expect their feelings to be part of a process where distress will eventually attenuate or resolve. However, if they are seen as necessarily being in need of intervention, the individual is helpless until the intervention is made available to them. Applied to communities or populations, significant numbers of people who are distressed as part of a normal psychological process come to see themselves as people who are ill and in need of help.

Summerfield believes that psychiatric concepts are culture-bound and ethnocentric. He highlights commentary in the psychiatric literature on refugees regarding the lack of psychological mindedness amongst non-Western populations. Refugees have to learn from Western mental health workers of their need for help. He points out that in contrast to this there is good evidence that the strongest moderating factors on the mental health of refugees are post-displacement social conditions and resolution of the conflict that caused displacement (Summerfield, 2008).

Within Summerfield's body of published work there is a suggestion that the assertion of an ever rising need for global mental health resources does not reflect an increase in the incidence of mental illnesses. Instead, an increase in demand for mental health care is a reflection of the spread of a culture that re-labels distress as illness and creates business opportunities for the mental health industry. Seen in this way, it becomes hard to know how valid international comparisons of the incidence of depression might be.

There is a critique of the conceptualisation of emotional distress as an illness that arises from within mainstream medicine and is similar to Healy's and Summerfield's (see for example Moynihan *et al.*, 2002). This critique does not attack the concept of mental illness; on the contrary, it rests on the assumption that there is a range of core conditions that are 'true' mental illnesses (such as schizophrenia, bipolar affective disorder and severe depression) which have essential features that differ from other forms of emotional suffering. However, the critique is severely critical of the application of the illness metaphor to non-illness conditions, such as bereavement, distress after involvement in traumatic events or minor and self-limiting day-to-day alterations in mood. According to this view, medicalising the problems of living undermines people's personal autonomy. It reduces the ability of the whole population to cope with the inevitable emotional turbulence of the human life cycle. It establishes an expectation of continuous happiness that is unrealistic. Thus the prescription of medication for non-illnesses or the provision of counselling for everyday distress is not only doomed to fail, it actually damages individuals and society as a whole, because people become dependent on professionals, medication and counselling to maintain their well-being.

The return of the mind–body dualism

Myalgic encephalopathy (ME) or chronic fatigue syndrome (CFS) is a condition of uncertain aetiology that causes considerable disability. One of the features is depression, and some researchers believe that it is, at least in part, psychological in origin (Wessely & Powell, 1989). This has led to huge controversy and anger. A significant proportion of people with ME consider the suggestion of a psychological aetiology to be an outrage (Hossenbaccus & White, 2013). To them, the idea is not just incorrect, it also trivialises their distress and suggests that the condition is inauthentic.

Self-help groups have organised and vociferously campaigned against the suggestion of a psychological cause. We do not suggest that they are necessarily wrong. However, here we have a contemporary movement, led by service users, that takes a position diametrically opposite to that of the anti-psychiatrists and post-psychiatrists. To ME activists, it is not the suggestion of *disease* that is stigmatising; it is the suggestion of an *absence of disease* that is problematic. The insistence that the psychological symptoms of the disorder are purely organic in origin places the logic of the ME lobby surprisingly close to the stereotypical biological psychiatrists' position; namely, that the relationship between the biological and the psychological is one of unidirectional causation, that neurotransmitter changes are of necessity causal of associated psychological changes. Indeed, there is a suggestion of an extrapolation to the position where suffering due to a physiological disturbance is regarded as more *authentic* than suffering due to a psychological disturbance.

Deconstructing psychiatric nosology

There have been attempts to deconstruct psychiatric nosology. In part, this has been an attempt to find new conceptual approaches to better understand mental disorder. In part, it has been ideological. Richard Bentall is one of the best known clinical psychologists conducting research into psychosis. Following a venerable tradition in experimental psychology, he has studied individual psychological symptoms or phenomena rather than whole syndromes (Bentall, 2004). This is a reasonable strategy, given that 100 years of research based upon the Kraeplinian nosological structure, which classifies psychosis into three large syndromes of dementia praecox/schizophrenia, manic-depression/bipolar affective disorder and paranoia/delusional disorder, has not led to any clarity over the fundamental nature of the psychoses.

Bentall is an empirical scientist who works within an assumption that psychotic symptoms are fundamentally organic rather than psychological in nature, but that they are better treated psychologically than physically (e.g. by the use of medication). He strongly objects to the concept of schizophrenia. Like Szasz, he believes that it is more an accusation than a true syndrome. Notoriously, he once published a paper lampooning psychiatric nosology by pointing out that happiness meets the criteria to be regarded as a mental disorder equally as well as, if not better than, traditional diagnoses such as schizophrenia (Bentall, 1992). This mischievously made point was reported in newspapers across the world as a serious attempt by psychiatrists to show that happiness was a mental abnormality. The paper found its way into a novel by Phillip Roth (Roth, 1996). Bentall cannot resist iconoclastic rhetoric, but his key scientific points have been increasingly absorbed into mainstream thinking. He has long held that psychosis is likely to be causally related to childhood adversity, whether social inequality or childhood sexual abuse. The evidence increasingly suggests that he is right. Notwithstanding his disdain for psychiatric diagnosis, he is closer to those who believe that social adversity causes mental illness than those who believe mental illness does not exist.

In defence of psychiatry

The fact that attacks on the concept of mental illness are so diverse, and often contradict each other, does not mean that they can be dismissed as incoherent. Organised psychiatry has continued to fight hard to retain a primarily biomedical understanding of mental disorder (Craddock *et al.*, 2008). Whether or not this is scientifically sustainable, there is an element of self-interest here. Doctors are by far the most privileged and best paid of all mental health professionals, and disease is their area of special expertise. If the disease model has little or no part in the understanding or treatment of mental distress, then the dominance of doctors is difficult to justify.

In the face of these various criticisms of the mental illness model, it is disappointing that we cannot identify a coherent and convincing defence of 'the medical model'. Two of us have taken the position that there is a medical model that has utility and is preferable to any of the alternatives at a practical level, but our work falls far short of a proper intellectual defence of the concept (Poole & Higgo, 2006). Broadly speaking, there are five main positions available, though there are many variations on these themes:
1. 'Mental illness' does not exist; it is a form of words used to marginalise behaviour that authority regards as undesirable.
2. Mental illness does exist, but isn't really illness or even necessarily undesirable. It is just another way of being. Living through it can lead to personal growth.
3. Emotional symptoms are caused by impersonal disease processes, not by psychological processes.
4. The symptoms of mental illness do exist, but they do not form illness syndromes.
5. Mental illness does exist, but only as discrete illness syndromes with clear boundaries. Other forms of human psychological suffering are not illnesses.

In our opinion, the weight of evidence suggests that the major mental illness syndromes do correspond to disease entities, and that their relationship with social deprivation is not tautologous. Our riposte to the argument (to borrow a phrase from Mandy Rice-Davies) 'well they would say that wouldn't they, two of them are psychiatrists' is that the evidence points to specific, if as yet poorly understood, social factors, which opens the possibility of effective preventative intervention.

Studying social factors and depression

There is a long history of research into depression and the social factors bearing upon individuals. This research first established that there are social antecedents to depressive symptoms. There were subsequent attempts to tease out the exact nature of the social factors that cause depression and those that protect against it.

Within the psychiatric literature there have been two broad common approaches to social factors. The first has utilised the concept of *life events*, whereby discrete occurrences (which might be positive or negative) are ranked according to perceived stressfulness, and for the degree of independence from the individual's own behaviour (i.e. bankruptcy is a dependent life event as it is contingent upon the person's behaviour. Being hit by a meteorite is an independent life event). The second approach has examined longer-term adverse social circumstances.

Paykel (2003) has reviewed the extensive evidence about life events and affective disorder. Most studies have been retrospective, comparing depressed subjects with non-depressed controls. There have also been studies of general population samples looking at rates of occurrence of life events and later onset of depressive symptoms. These studies have shown a consistent association between life events and depressive symptoms. A variety of events are involved, with no particular pattern with regard to the meaning of events, other than a larger effect due to threatening or undesirable events. Life events affect remission and relapse in affective disorder, but they are less important in recurrent and severe illness.

There is an association between bipolar disorder and life events, particularly at first onset, but it is weaker than for unipolar depression. However, bipolar disorder is hard to study in life-event research, owing to the relatively high rate of dependent life events relating to mania and its consequences. There is a stronger association between life events and depression than schizophrenia. Suicide attempts are more strongly associated with life events than depression without self-harm. Life events have a clearer impact on depressive symptoms where there are co-morbidities such as substance dependence. Life events are important in all age groups. Interestingly, antecedent life events are no less common where the clinical presentation is melancholia than for other depressions.

Studies of long-term social factors in depression have produced well-known findings. Brown and Harris published a seminal book in 1978 based upon an extensive programme of research on the social factors associated with depression in a community sample of women living in Camberwell (Brown & Harris, 1978). This showed that being an unemployed working-class single mother looking after small children in the absence of a confiding relationship was highly predictive of depressive symptoms. The finding was not surprising. It drew out social origins of depression in a particular population of women, without necessarily illuminating the social origins of depression in general. One of the criticisms of this work was that it was far from clear that the participating women were suffering from syndromal depression as opposed to depressive symptoms or ordinary human unhappiness.

There is a body of work in social science that understands the impact of social adversity in terms of broad social networks, rather than as isolated phenomena affecting individuals. Rosenquist and colleagues examined the clustering of depressed individuals within social networks (Rosenquist *et al.*, 2011). They used data from the Framingham heart study, a large long-term cohort study, to examine network connections between people suffering from depression. They showed

that there was clustering of moderately and severely depressed individuals. They identified three possible mechanisms that might cause this:
1. depression in one person induces depression in others;
2. depressed individuals seek each other out;
3. confounding, whereby connected individuals are subject to the same social environment with the same results.

Depressed individuals were more likely than others to exist at the periphery of their social network. Clustering was evident up to three degrees of separation and disappeared at four; in other words, clustering did not depend on direct social contact between depressed individuals, but did depend on a degree of social proximity.

Social networks had an impact on relapse. People with more friends and social ties were less likely to experience further depression in the future. However, the number of family members had no effect. People who were depressed on average lost 6% of their friends over a four-year period, whereas people who were not depressed increased the number of their friends over time. However, it was the proportion of the individual's social network that was depressed that had an effect upon them rather than the absolute number of people in the network. Depression spreads more easily than lack of depression (i.e. the protective effect of having non-depressed individuals in a social network was of a smaller magnitude than the negative effect of having depressed individuals within it). Depression spreads more easily *from* women than *from* men. However, it spreads *to* both genders with equal ease. The evidence from this study is that social networks affect the occurrence of depression, but social networks are affected by the individual's mental health. There are some echoes of Durkheim in the findings as isolation has a discernible effect, those with fewer social contacts being more easily affected.

Social capital

This work on social networks is the converse of the ideas concerning social capital discussed in Chapter 2. Here is an example of the way in which social networks can be vectors for social stress and disadvantage. Social capital is a model of social networks as vectors of social resilience. Social networks are not necessarily based upon localities. However, it may be that social networks that are based around deprived areas carry little social capital and therefore lack a protective function with regard to mental health (Haines *et al.*, 2011).

There has been recent work that attempts to measure directly the impact of social capital on depression (Webber *et al.*, 2011). Depressed people with more social capital showed no greater improvement over six months than those with less social capital. What did make a difference was the quality of supportive emotional relationships, which the authors point out supports the Brown and Harris model where confiding relationships are one of the critical factors in protecting against depression. It is arguable that the problem with this literature is that it reifies social capital to the point where meaning is squeezed out of social relationships.

The large body of research on social factors and depression eventually brings us to a frustratingly inconclusive place. Depression is certainly affected by a range of social factors, most of which are associated with a lack of financial resources. Although psychiatrists rarely speak of endogenous depression any more, there is a case for the validity of the category. Melancholia does appear to have the features of a disease entity. Whilst the first onset of depression is closely related to life events, established recurrent severe depression is much less influenced by them. There is a marked tautological flavour to the finding that living in bad social circumstances generates misery. What is striking, however, is the complete lack of evidence that the experience of grappling with social adversity confers any benefit or protection against depression. 'That which does not destroy me makes me strong' is a statement that runs contrary to the evidence.

The Happiness Agenda

As long ago as 1980, the economist Richard (now Lord) Layard suggested that economic growth and increasing national wealth in the UK was not leading to greater levels of happiness (Layard, 1980). Layard has subsequently had an enormous impact on mental health policy in the UK.

Layard takes the view that the primary responsibility of government is to increase the amount of happiness in society. Although this idea has a certain appeal because it sounds like a truism, it is far from self-evident. Within social science, it is an idea that belongs to modern radical liberalism. It stands in opposition to neo-conservative ideas (that the role of the state is solely to facilitate commerce), older liberal ideas (that the role of government is to safeguard social justice and fairness) and Marxist ideas (that government represents class interest). Layard summarised many of his ideas in the Lionel Robbins Memorial Lectures.[2] According to him, happiness is the most important good. Happiness means feeling good, enjoying life and feeling that life is wonderful. Unhappiness means feeling bad and wishing things were different. Happiness and unhappiness are on a single continuum. Layard appears to see no real distinction between unhappiness and depression. To him, unhappiness is a mental health issue.

As an economist, Layard discusses his ideas from a distinctively economic viewpoint. However, he has a strong interest in psychology and neuroscience. He draws upon concepts and data from those disciplines to substantiate his point of view. He presents evidence to show that on an individual level, in the short term, a rise in income is associated with an increase in happiness. However, in the longer term, the individual's happiness fades due to habituation. The effect of a rise in income

---

[2] Layard R (2003) Happiness: Has social science a clue? Lionel Robbins Memorial Lecture 2003 www. stoa.org.uk/topics/happiness/ *retrieved 28 November 2012.*

for one person is to reduce the happiness of others owing to rivalry. He proposes that taxation policy should be adjusted to create an optimum work/life balance which would maximise happiness across the whole population. He recognises that this might lead to a reduction in Gross Domestic Product (GDP), but notes that GDP is not equivalent to happiness or necessarily associated with it.

Layard had a number of other proposals for making society happier. These included measures related to work, work-related stress, and job security. Other measures included policies to promote security for families and communities, policies for mental health, and policies to promote personal and political freedom. He suggested that participatory democracy should be promoted, but he did not have any specific proposals in this regard. He did not explain how this would lead to greater happiness. He believed that mental health should have a higher priority within social policy, meaning that public spending on mental health should be higher.

Writing in 2007, Layard and his colleagues (Layard *et al.*, 2007) commented on the high proportion of the population who suffer from what they labelled 'severe mental illness'. This did not correspond to the use of the term within mental health services or the psychiatric literature, where it is mainly used as a synonym for psychotic illnesses. They repeated the widely cited statistic that 25% of adults suffer from a mental health problem at some point in their lives, with 16% suffering from anxiety or depression. Mental illness was described as causing as much misery as poverty does. In keeping with this statement, there is a tendency in much of Layard's work to discuss mental illness as if it were independent of poverty and other social factors, except in so far as mental illness impairs productivity. In other words, Layard seems to believe that causality runs from mental illness to poverty.

Layard and his colleagues stated that the means existed to treat mental illness effectively. These were set out in the relevant National Institute for Health and Care Excellence (NICE) guidance. However, NICE guidance could not be implemented to full effect, as at that time spending on mental health services was insufficient. They stated that cognitive behaviour therapy (CBT) was a particularly effective treatment, but that far too few trained CBT therapists were available. They claimed that if there was a major programme over 5 to 10 years, therapists could be trained and deployed in therapy centres, and that this would significantly reduce the overall burden of mental ill health within British society. The result would be a major improvement in the level of happiness in the UK population.

The authors made an economic case for their proposals. They claimed that a large programme to make CBT available to those unable to work could reduce the number of people on incapacity benefit. The programme would get them back to work, with benefits for the individual and society as a whole. They projected a cost saving to society of £19,400 over a two-year period for each person successfully treated. This was made up of savings in direct benefit payments of £18,000, an increase in GDP of £1,100 and a saving to the NHS of £300. The cost of a course of CBT was calculated to be £750. Recovery rates of 50% of those treated were anticipated. On this basis, the programme would be self-funding, even if a significant proportion of people treated did not recover.

Layard's proposals had a mixed response within the mental health professions. On the one hand, it was generally accepted that access to effective psychological therapies was poor, especially amongst those who could not afford private therapy. On the other hand, there was scepticism that it was possible to produce a major change in public health through a programme of individual intervention, particularly as the programme and interventions appeared to take little account of the social context in which long-term invalidism due to anxiety and depression occurred. The proposals were very appealing to the New Labour government of the time, which had no fixed political ideology but a strong attachment to extrapolating experimental evidence into major social policies.

Layard's therapy programme was implemented in stages from 2006 as the IAPT initiative. Two pilot sites were chosen, in Doncaster and Newham, with an associated evaluation (Clark et al., 2008). The evaluation was quasi-experimental and a number of assumptions had to be made. During the time of the study 5,500 people were referred and 3,500 concluded their involvement with the services. One third had had their problems for six months or less, and one third for more than two years. Nineteen hundred people had two or more treatment sessions, 52% of people were said to have made a good recovery but no figures were provided for the anticipated rate of recovery without intervention. Five per cent of people completing treatment secured jobs, and the overall employment rate increased by 4%.

There were far more participants in Doncaster than in Newham. In the detailed figures for Doncaster, of 4,451 referrals, 378 were judged unsuitable for therapy as they had high symptom scores, perhaps because they were too ill to benefit from CBT. Eight hundred and seventy-seven were suitable but received no treatment, and 571 attended once only. No data were presented on quality of life or functioning. For cases of less than six months' duration, the outcome was no different to the recovery rate assumed by the authors in the absence of intervention. The figures suggest that very few people receive a full course of treatment, that there is a high dropout rate, and that many of the people referred had problems of short duration and would have recovered spontaneously.

There have been further evaluations of IAPT, but the costs and actual recovery rates remain unclear. Radhakrishnan and colleagues (Radhakrishnan et al., 2013) studied the cost of the treatment and recovery rates in selected Primary Care Trusts in the East of England. They calculated an average cost per session of £137.73. High-intensity cases cost £176.97 per session. They assumed natural or spontaneous recovery rates of 30% and claimed that treatment through IAPT increased that by 20%.

So far, it has not been convincingly demonstrated that IAPT is making progress towards its objectives. For example, assessment of the effects of IAPTs differ according to whether intention-to-treat analyses are taken from the point that a general practitioner (GP) refers the patient to an IAPT team, or from the point at which they are accepted for treatment. We believe that intention-to-treat should be taken from the point of referral. Analysis based on this starting point makes IAPT look less effective and more expensive than some reports have suggested.

A key assumption that was used to justify investment in IAPT was that it would improve social functioning and promote return to work. The NICE guidance on which IAPT is based cites research that measures outcome mainly through changes in symptom ratings rather than in terms of changes in quality of life or social functioning. The assumption that symptom ratings, quality of life and social functioning are closely related is questionable. A review of the studies cited by NICE examined those studies that did use quality of life and functioning outcomes. Interpersonal therapy (IPT) and CBT were not effective by those measures (McPherson *et al.*, 2009).

IAPT was rolled out across England prior to the publication of the results of the evaluation of the pilots. It is hard to know how successful the project has been, in part because the credit crunch of 2008 and the subsequent economic recession has obscured any progress that might have been achieved. However, there are key problems with IAPT as a large-scale intervention to improve the mental health of the nation:

Firstly, in practice IAPT teams have tended to be swamped with referrals. It is well recognised that 20% of GP consultations relate to mental health concerns. The existence of a service to address these needs without recourse to medication has encouraged referral, notwithstanding the fact that many of the problems referred would have resolved without intervention. The pressures caused by processing large numbers of referrals has meant that interventions tend to be brief or very brief.

Secondly, investment in IAPT has occurred at a time when core services for people with psychotic illness have been under severe financial pressure. Many mental health professionals have felt that service priorities have been skewed away from people with serious problems towards the 'worried well'. Although Layard has conflated mental illness, depression and unhappiness, it is far from clear that this is valid. In our opinion, it is certain that it is not.

Thirdly, the economic success of IAPT depends on people experiencing a functional recovery in response to CBT. However, large numbers of people on invalidity benefit have complex problems and these are unlikely to respond well to basic CBT techniques.

Fourthly, there are very few, if any, examples of treatments at the individual level resulting in an improvement in public health. For example, vaccination programmes are successful not because they treat diseased individuals, but because they increase herd immunity.

Finally, Layard originally proposed mental health intervention as part of a much larger programme of change, which included structural economic change. If depression and anxiety are to any substantial extent a consequence of poverty and other social adversity, it is highly unlikely that it will be possible to reduce their prevalence without action to address underlying causes.

Main points in this chapter

1. Modern critiques of the medicalisation of distress ('disease-mongering') have credibility. They dictate caution in assuming that responses to adversity are necessarily pathological.
2. Affective disorder syndromes such as bipolar affective disorder and melancholia are different to ordinary emotional distress. They are affected by social factors.
3. There is a substantial body of work demonstrating a link between life events and affective disorders, although these are less important in chronic and severe illnesses.
4. Long-term social factors are relevant to affective disorders.
5. IAPT is a large-scale experimental effort to improve the happiness of the population of England. It is far from clear that it has been successful.

5

Genetics

Genetic determinism is a thread in Western thinking that has a long history, although it was conceptualised as *hereditary taint* until the twentieth century. It has been influential in intellectual traditions far beyond the scientific. It can be detected in politics, in literature and in everyday concepts of individuality. There is a commonplace interaction that greatly discomforts teenagers at family events, whereby every physical and temperamental characteristic that they possess is attributed to the hereditary legacy of some relative (often long-deceased) or another. This folk concept is hard to resist, and even those of us who should know better sometimes indulge it. However, it is based on a misapprehension concerning fundamental genetic processes. In fact, the genetic machinery recombines genes in as many ways as possible, in order to produce individuals with a great diversity of overall phenotype, each of which is unique to them (except in the cases of monozygotic twins). Far from being trapped by the combined effects of hereditary and family environment, human beings display an extraordinary range of personal characteristics that are emergent and cannot be so easily explained.

There is a massive literature on the genetics of mental illness. For a substantial proportion of psychiatrists, the debate over the role of genes in major mental illness was settled decades ago in favour of the biological. In contrast, we have presented evidence that suggests that environmental factors not only precipitate and shape mental illness, but that they might have a significant causal role. There is a problem with a model where a hermetically sealed genotype interacts with the environment to produce a behavioural phenotype. There are contradictions between different bodies of knowledge that are difficult to reconcile. In this chapter we examine this issue, and draw out some of the complexities of studying gene–environment interaction with reference to the example of cannabis and schizophrenia.

Mental illness and genes

Since the nineteenth century, psychiatry has held that there is a hereditary element to major mental illness. This is definitely correct for some diseases that lead to gross cerebral pathology. For example, a great deal is known about the specific genetic factors that cause Huntington's disease. The condition is an important exemplar where molecular genetics have allowed epidemiological, clinical, pathological and genetic evidence to be tied together to create an overall understanding.

Huntington's disease can manifest itself at any age, but it most commonly causes symptoms in early middle age. Initial symptoms tend to be change in personality, psychiatric symptoms and subtle alterations in cognitive function. Over time, the condition steadily worsens, with the development of dementia and neurological symptoms such as choreiform movements. A particular feature of the condition is agitation and distress. It has long been recognised that Huntington's disease follows a Mendelian dominant pattern of inheritance. Offspring have a 50% chance of inheriting the gene and hence of developing the condition.

People with Huntington's disease produce large quantities of an abnormal form of a protein, Huntingtin, which is deposited in body tissues. It causes problems in the brain and it damages other tissues. Everyone has Huntingtin present in their body, but in modest amounts and in a non-mutated form. The disorder is caused by an abnormal number of trinucleotide repeats on a section of a specific gene, the HTT gene, located on the short arm of chromosome 4. The abnormal repeat sequence is cytosine–adenine–guanine (CAG), which codes for the amino acid glutamine. When people have more than 36 CAG repeats in the gene, they manifest Huntington's disease. The genetic abnormality leads to more repeat sequences being present in each successive generation, with more rapid deposition of Huntingtin and earlier and more severe symptoms. A gene probe has been developed that allows people to know whether they have the condition before they show symptoms.

This demonstrates the potential of molecular genetics. The genetic abnormality can be tied to the production of an abnormal protein with specific pathological effects on the body, causing corresponding symptoms that follow an understandable course and outcome. The gene probe is of diagnostic value, and the possibility exists of eventually being able to intervene biochemically.

The picture for psychotic illnesses is much more complex. Genetic evidence on the major functional disorders continues to accumulate at a staggering rate, but the knowledge acquired so far does not paint a coherent picture. There have been numerous claims of an imminent breakthrough over many years. So far, a breakthrough to treatment has not occurred and the precise nature of genetic risk in these disorders remains elusive. Some recent findings suggest that the fundamental premise on which the promise of a breakthrough is based is false, at least with regard to the prospect of answers similar to those found for Huntington's disease.

All psychiatrists are familiar with the research techniques and evidence that underlie the belief that schizophrenia and bipolar disorder are predominantly genetic conditions, modulated by environmental factors (for example, see Tsuang *et al.*, 2001). Taken together, family studies, adoption studies and twin studies create a formidable body of evidence that is often summarised in the statement that schizophrenia is 80% heritable, with environmental factors of all sorts accounting for just 20% of variance. However, the assertion that there is a fixed percentage of causation attributable to genetic factors in conditions where both genes and the environment play a role is fallacious.

Take smoking and lung cancer as an example. In societies where some people smoke, but many people do not, the vast majority of cases of lung cancer will occur amongst smokers. The condition can be regarded as overwhelmingly due to an environmental factor, smoking. However, in a society where everybody smoked 20 a day, the biggest factor determining who developed lung cancer and who did not would be genetic susceptibility. The 80:20 formula is seriously misleading with regard to the degree to which the incidence might be modifiable by changing the environment in which people live.

There is clear empirical evidence which shows that where measurable psychological characteristics are determined by both genes and environment, alteration of the environment has significant effects. There is a body of work on intelligence that demonstrates this. To take just one example, working-class children adopted into middle-class families show a significant increase in IQ (Nisbett et al., 2012). Similar findings have emerged for most of the mental disorders where both environmental factors and genetic factors appear to be of importance. In recent times, researchers in biological psychiatry have started to acknowledge that the primacy of genetic factors is not as secure or overwhelming as they have sometimes suggested in the past.

We do not advocate genetic denial. It would be very surprising to find any human characteristic or vulnerability where genetics were irrelevant. Our species is undeniably structurally programmed by genes, and genetic diversity in the human population is pervasive and obvious. The nature versus nurture debates of the mid twentieth century were ultimately barren and unproductive, because they dichotomised evidence that was better understood in its totality. Until recently, psychiatry was stuck in the residuum of that debate, and the emergence of a more balanced understanding is a significant step forward.

Much of the genetic research in psychiatry conducted over the past 30 years has been focussed on identifying candidate genes that might confer psychotic vulnerability, analogous to the situation with Huntington's disease. At present, opinion favours a likely multitude of genes of small effect, although the single genetic lesion model has not disappeared. However, the fundamental evidence for the heritability of schizophrenia and other major mental illnesses does not depend on molecular genetics. It rests upon epidemiology and studies of risk using either administrative data sets or clinical studies of the relatives of affected individuals. This research is not easy to conduct, and there are numerous methodological pitfalls, such as case definition and ascertainment.

In 2009, the findings of a record linkage study of the entire population of Sweden (Lichtenstein et al., 2009) suggested that schizophrenia and bipolar affective disorder are not genetically separate. The authors suggested an additive genetic model. In the same year, the International Schizophrenia Consortium published a genome-wide study in the journal *Nature* (International Schizophrenia Consortium, 2009) where statistical criteria were relaxed in order to investigate the contribution of more than a thousand genes of small effect. The authors created sum scores for polygenic associations. The genes in question appeared to account for 30% of the variance in the risk of developing schizophrenia and bipolar disorder in the 7,000 participants included in the study. More recently, a paper in the *Lancet* (Cross-Disorder Group of the Psychiatric Genetics Consortium, 2013) has suggested that syndromic approaches to diagnosis may not be valid and that it might be better to define disorders genetically. This is based on the finding that four gene loci, two of which relate to calcium channel activity, have an effect on five different disorders, namely autism spectrum disorder, attention deficit-hyperactivity disorder, bipolar affective disorder, major depressive disorder and schizophrenia.

In the light of challenging genetic evidence like this, combined with strong evidence about the importance of social factors in most forms of mental illness, psychiatry has at last started to move away from genetic determinism. This has been unhelpful in the past and it has ultimately proven scientifically unsustainable. Professor Sir Robin Murray is one of the most distinguished schizophrenia researchers in the world. Much of his work has been biological, though over the past decade he has increasingly investigated environmental factors. Recently he has acknowledged that genetic (or biological) determinism has been destructive to both the science and practice of psychiatry.[1]

Socio-biology

Socio-biology is a modern extrapolation of genetic determinism. The central tenet is that social behaviour, and therefore society itself, is determined by biological factors, which a priori are ultimately genetic. This has been highly controversial ever since the doctrine was first clearly articulated in the 1970s (Wilson, 1975; Lewontin *et al.*, 1984). The best known of the contemporary advocates of socio-biology is Richard Dawkins, who set out a particular version of it in his book *The Selfish Gene* (Dawkins, 1976). Dawkins' contribution to genetics has been to promote the view that natural selection and evolution can best be understood in terms of individual genes, not individual organisms or populations. Genes have only two fundamental characteristics, one of which is to determine a phenotype and the other of which is replication. Genes persist in populations because they replicate and pass on to subsequent generations. They can only do this if they enhance survival of the individual organism that carries them. This much makes sense. It is not contradicted by the persistence of harmful recessive genes or by the lack of evidence that all human characteristics are determined by individual single genes.

[1] For example www.schizophreniacommission.org.uk/2012/03/professor-sir-robin-murray-on-bbc-radio-4/ *retrieved 29 May 2013.*

However, Dawkins extrapolates to a position that all characteristics of organisms *of necessity* must be genetically determined and must be subject to selective pressures. In this argument, altruism and the tendency to form cooperative social groupings are expressions of gene function and they serve a gene survival purpose. To Dawkins this is a truism, but to the sceptical it is highly contentious. We accept a similar materialistic understanding of existence to Dawkins, but his rigidly mechanistic causal pathway from the molecular to the social seems to us to be unsustainable. It is possible to construct convoluted arguments in support of his position so that, for example, the wisdom of old age or the appreciation of artistic beauty might carry a single gene propagation advantage. It seems to us to be far more likely that many human characteristics emerge as a consequence of the way humans live and interact. They may have a relationship to our genetic blueprint but they are not necessarily determined by it. Furthermore, it is likely that genes, constantly recombining, interact with each other in ways that produce particular attributes that have significant consequences for phenotype, but which may not be subject to selective pressure. This seems to us to be a scientifically robust position. Dawkins' assertion of a single universal mechanism that controls everything has an explanatory power similar to the concept of the controlling hand of a deity. Like intelligent design, it currently lacks either evidence or refutability.

Gene–environment interaction: schizophrenia and cannabis

For a decade there was a plethora of publications in the scientific journals on the relationship between cannabis use and schizophrenia. There was much public concern, a high level of media coverage, and there were changes to the British law. There are a number of lessons to be drawn from this controversy. There was an interesting false dawn where for a moment it appeared that the influence of an environmental factor could be related to a single trinucleotide polymorphism at a specific gene locus.

It has been known since the nineteenth century that psychotic illness is associated with substance misuse. Modern findings confirm that people with schizophrenia and bipolar affective disorder are more likely than the general population to be heavy users of tobacco, alcohol and cannabis. Most studies suggest that amongst people diagnosed with schizophrenia roughly 30% misuse alcohol and 15–30% misuse drugs. The drug most commonly used is cannabis. Rates of opiate use amongst people diagnosed with schizophrenia have never been found to be much higher than the rate amongst the general population. A proportion misuse both alcohol and cannabis, so that roughly 50% of people with schizophrenia misuse one or other substance. The term 'dual diagnosis' has been widely applied to these patients. However, the term is a logical nonsense. There are many other possible 'dual diagnoses' alongside schizophrenia, for example, learning disability. More importantly, if half of everyone with schizophrenia has a substance misuse problem, and if this is much higher than the general population prevalence, then substance misuse should be properly regarded as an intrinsic part of the schizophrenia syndrome. There is no need to invoke a second diagnosis, which only causes confusion.

Cannabis contains a potent mixture of psychoactive substances with complex effects. In Europe, cannabis is generally regarded as a calming drug with mildly psychedelic effects. In other cultures and at other times it has had different reputations, for example as an analgesic or even as an enhancer of aggression. The term 'assassin' is said to derive from the word 'hashish', which was allegedly used by notoriously fierce warriors in Afghanistan and Pakistan prior to doing battle. Cannabis contains as many as 50 pharmacologically active substances, some of which are cannabinoids, and some of which are found in other plant species. Isbell and colleagues carried out classic experimental work on the pharmacology of the drug in the 1960s (Isbell *et al.*, 1967). Trans-Δ^9-tetrahydrocannabinol (Δ^9-THC) was identified as the most potent cannabinoid, with actions that are typical of the widely recognised psychological effects of cannabis intoxication. In due course, cannabinoid receptors were identified in the human brain. Isbell's 1967 paper described one individual who experienced a paranoid reaction on administration of Δ^9-THC. Other cannabinoids have only started to be studied in detail relatively recently. For example, cannabidiol appears to have antipsychotic properties in addition to its known anticonvulsant effects (Morgan & Curran, 2008).

The concentration of cannabinoids in cannabis plants is dependent on the subspecies and the conditions that the plant is exposed to whilst it is growing. It is particularly dependent on exposure to ultraviolet light. Cannabinoids oxidise readily in air. Commercial cannabis producers grow high Δ^9-THC-yield varieties in hydroponic systems under optimal climatic and lighting conditions. Much of the cannabis that is consumed in the UK is produced locally in cannabis factories with rapid distribution to end users. In contrast, until the 1980s most cannabis was imported into the UK in the form of resin. This was produced in North Africa and the Middle East by compressing flowering tops of hemp plants. Importation and distribution was relatively slow, and during these lengthy processes cannabinoids in the resin oxidised owing to prolonged exposure to air. As a consequence of changes in production and distribution, cannabis sold in the UK today is two to three times stronger in Δ^9-THC than the resin that was available 30 years ago. There are specialist preparations that are stronger still. However, the concept of 'skunk' and 'super skunk' (i.e. a type of generally available super cannabis with qualitatively different effects to old-fashioned resinous hashish) was a marketing concept that was earnestly adopted in a moral panic by the UK media. Newspapers became convinced that there was a new type of cannabis available with unique and dangerous effects. Whilst it is true that cannabis is readily and cheaply available throughout the UK, it is not true that this represents a new danger. The issue of strength is a red herring. It is believed that cannabis users, like smokers addicted to nicotine, adjust their consumption of different strengths to achieve a relatively stable preferred level of intoxication (Select Committee on Science and Technology, 1998). Cannabis supply has for some years been at saturation point in the UK.

Cannabis is so cheap and so freely available that for all intents and purposes most people can use as much as they like without compromising their finances.

In 1996, a paper reviewing the concept of drug-induced psychosis (Poole & Brabbins, 1996) noted a single study published nine years earlier that showed an association between self-reported cannabis use on conscription to the Swedish army and later diagnosis of schizophrenia (Andreasson *et al.*, 1987). The review paper suggested that the finding might be a consequence of neglected confounding factors associated with both early cannabis use and schizophrenia. This provoked an aggrieved response from the authors of the Swedish conscript study that they had controlled for a variety of factors, including social class (Allebeck & Andreasson, 1996).

From the early 2000s there was intense scientific interest in the relationship between cannabis use and schizophrenia, with a flood of publications on the subject, which continues unabated at the time of writing. A systematic review (Moore *et al.*, 2007) published in the *Lancet* in 2007 concluded that the literature up to that time demonstrated that individuals who had ever used cannabis had an increased risk of developing psychosis (pooled adjusted Odds Ratio = 1.4, 95% Confidence Interval 1.20–1.65) and that there was a dose response effect, with the heaviest users carrying a greater risk (Odds Ratio 2.09, CI 1.54–2.84). Subsequently, some authoritative researchers in this area have asserted that, notwithstanding some acknowledged ambiguities in the evidence, the causal role of cannabis in schizophrenia is established beyond reasonable doubt and that the public should be warned. This view has been highly influential. Although the government's advisory body (the Advisory Committee on the Misuse of Drugs) was not convinced by the evidence for a causal relationship between cannabis use and schizophrenia, in 2009 their advice (that change to the law on cannabis was not justified) was ignored. Penalties for possession and distribution of cannabis had been downgraded in 2004, when it was reclassified from a class B to a class C drug. This was reversed in 2009 under the influence of lobbying that cannabis use was an avoidable cause of schizophrenia. The change was predicated upon a belief that the legal classification of cannabis might somehow reduce users' consumption, and hence reduce the incidence of schizophrenia in the UK.

The issue about the role of confounding factors in studying the relationship between cannabis use in teenagers and the later development of schizophrenia was somewhat misunderstood in the 1996 riposte by the authors of the Swedish study. Not just anyone smokes cannabis heavily in their early teens. It is a behaviour that is associated with a range of other problems and with social deprivation in particular. These other problems are known to be associated with an increased risk of schizophrenia, and thus early heavy cannabis use could be acting as a marker of risk rather than as a causal factor per se. These confounding factors are not easy to control for. In the Swedish conscript study, the measures that were used were relatively crude and may not have eliminated the impact of factors independently associated with both schizophrenia and early cannabis use. All of the major studies on cannabis and schizophrenia have attempted to control for confounding factors.

However, the credibility of the conclusion that cannabis has an established role in the causation of schizophrenia does depend upon adequate adjustment in order to rid findings of significant confounding effects. In assessing this, it is necessary to add some caveats.

Anyone can pull research apart, as is clearly demonstrated on a regular basis in journal clubs in academic departments of psychiatry throughout the country. If one sets impossibly high standards of methodological perfection, then little research will be conducted and knowledge will not progress. There is always a difficult judgement to be made as to when sufficiently robust evidence has accumulated to regard a hypothesis to be proven or an association to be causal. The need for this type of judgement is a feature of most science. It is codified in setting the threshold of significance at 5%, for example, in the use of 95% confidence intervals, which simply reflects what most people regard as a reasonable level of certainty. Cannabis is a drug that can have unpleasant effects and that has particularly damaging consequences for people who suffer from a mental illness. The scientific question about the cannabis and schizophrenia findings is whether sufficient has been done to exclude alternative explanations for findings other than direct causality.

In 2006, the *British Medical Journal* published a brief review regarding the evidence concerning cannabis and psychosis (Fergusson *et al.*, 2006). It mentioned the possibility that there were residual uncontrolled confounding factors in recent large epidemiological studies, but pointed out that these had controlled for a wide range of factors, including sex, age, previous mental health problems (particularly psychosis prior to cannabis use), educational level, personality, IQ, association with deviant peers, conduct and attention disorders, other substance misuse, social functioning, parental factors, parental offending and substance misuse, socio-economic factors, physical and sexual abuse, and childhood trauma. This is a fairly comprehensive range of factors, which taken together might be reasonably expected to vicariously control for the effects of, for example, growing up in urban deprivation. However, different studies controlled for different factors. They involved participants included through varying criteria, using different methods. The fact that the studies taken as a group controlled for a wide range of confounding factors does not necessarily mean that each individual study eliminated confounding factors in general or a link with urban deprivation in particular. It is at least theoretically possible that each study inadequately controlled for one or more confounding factors, producing an aggregated confounded finding.

The first of these studies (Zammit *et al.*, 2002), which was published in 2002, was an extension of the 1987 Swedish conscript study. Like the original study, it took information that had been routinely collected from Swedish men when they were conscripted into the army in 1969–1970 at the age of 18–20. Only 3% of Swedish men were excused conscription, mainly because of physical or learning disability. The cohort was large, comprising 50,087 men. Each conscript completed a series of detailed self-administered questionnaires. There were psychological and physical evaluations of each of the men. Rates of missing data were very low. Information was linked to the Swedish national hospital discharge register in order to detect admissions with a diagnosis of schizophrenia. The purpose of this second study was to extend the follow-up period (originally 15 years, now 27 years) and to eliminate possible confounding factors that had not been controlled in the 1987 study. Those participants with a diagnosis of schizophrenia at the time of conscription were excluded.

In the analysis, logistic regression was used to calculate Odds Ratios for being admitted with International Classification of Disease, 8th and 9th Editions (ICD-8 or ICD-9) schizophrenia, comparing participants who admitted to cannabis use with those who denied it. The paper reported unadjusted Odds Ratios alongside Odds Ratios after adjustment for confounding factors. The following were regarded as potential confounders in the analysis: psychiatric diagnosis at conscription; IQ; personality variables (derived from questions about social behaviour); place of upbringing; paternal age; cigarette smoking; disturbed behaviour in childhood; history of alcohol misuse; family history of psychiatric illness; family's financial situation; father's occupation.

The original 1987 study had shown a 6 times increased risk of schizophrenia for those who admitted to cannabis use, which reduced to 2.7 times when participants who had been already diagnosed with a mental illness at the time of conscription were excluded. The heaviest cannabis users had a 3% risk of being diagnosed with schizophrenia in the next 15 years. The 2002 study, with longer follow-up and greater attention to confounding factors, confirmed the previous findings. The unadjusted Odds Ratio for cannabis users was 6.7. Adjusting for potential confounding factors reduced the Odds Ratio to 2.3. However, many of the potential confounders appeared to have little effect on the results. The ones that did were low IQ, urban childhood, early disturbed behaviour, cigarette smoking and poor social integration. These are all factors associated with inner-city deprivation. Their combined effect was larger than the effect of cannabis use.

The method of assessing these factors may not have been sufficiently sensitive to eliminate a residual confounding effect. For example, urban childhood is known to confer an increased risk. We have seen in earlier chapters that amongst people with an urban childhood there is a far larger effect of growing up in very deprived areas, and a relatively small or non-existent effect of growing up in wealthy suburbs. If heavy early cannabis use is also associated with growing up in very deprived areas, lumping together everyone with an urban birth may not be sufficient to fully control for the effect of a significant confounding factor. It is a matter of judgement as to whether issues of this kind are likely to have had an effect of sufficient magnitude to account for the whole of the apparent association between early cannabis use and later schizophrenia.

A group led by Jim van Os published findings on the effects of cannabis in 2002 (Van Os *et al.*, 2002). This study was part of the Netherlands Mental Health Survey and Incidence Study (NEMESIS). A random sample of 7,076 Dutch residents were contacted and interviewed at home by non-clinician researchers, who supervised the completion of a self-administered questionnaire. Participants were contacted again one year and three years later, with a similar procedure. Participants who described any psychotic symptoms at baseline were re-interviewed over the telephone by a research psychiatrist using a structured validated diagnostic interview schedule. At three-year follow-up there was a further psychiatric telephone interview using different symptom rating scales.

As is usual in this type of study, there was a high rate of attrition. Of the original sample, 4,848 participants completed the study. The authors made appropriate statistical analyses to estimate the effect of attrition on the results. Although the number of participants was large, as a sample of the general population it was small. The follow-up period was relatively brief. It was inevitable that the number of participants who developed psychosis in the follow-up period was small. Of the 4,045 participants who reported no psychotic symptoms at any time in their lives at baseline, seven had psychotic symptoms suggesting a definite or probable need for treatment three years later. A further 48 participants had psychotic symptoms at lower intensities not requiring care.

Cannabis use at baseline was associated with psychotic symptoms at all levels after three years. This remained true after adjustment for age, sex, ethnic group, marital status, educational attainment, urbanicity and level of discrimination. Urbanicity was measured at three levels of intensity rather than two as in the Swedish study. The Odds Ratio for cannabis use at baseline and psychotic symptoms after three years was very high, 23.32, but the confidence intervals were wide, which was a consequence of the small numbers affected. For frank psychotic illness in need of treatment, the population attributable fraction was 50%. In other words, within the limitations of the study, if cannabis was assumed to have played a causal role, half of these individuals would not have become psychotic if they had not used cannabis.

The study convincingly confirms the association between prior cannabis use and later psychotic symptoms. The main problem with the paper is the small number of people developing frank psychotic illness. The paper, in keeping with other work by Jim van Os, makes the assumption that psychotic symptoms lie on a continuum that ranges from isolated single symptoms to frank psychotic illness. To Van Os, low-level symptoms, such as auditory hallucinations, reflect a vulnerability to psychotic breakdown, or *forme fruste* psychosis. It is not self-evident that this is correct, and there are cogent arguments to the contrary. Large numbers of people have low-level experiences of this sort, including people with borderline personality disorder and people with a charismatic religious faith. It is entirely possible that their experiences arise through different mechanisms to those that are associated with full-blown psychotic illness.

If one ignores the participants with sub-clinical psychotic symptoms, an association remains. As is the case in the Swedish conscript study, it is plausible that there was a residual confounding effect and that even the three-intensity-level approach to urbanicity used in the study was insufficient to eliminate it. The judgement, as before, is whether a residual confounding effect could be large enough to produce such a large Odds Ratio. If one ignores the sub-clinical group and concentrates on the seven people with psychosis, then the answer is definitely yes because of the small sample size. The riposte by those who disagree with us would be that these findings have to be seen in the context of the rest of the literature, and on this we agree.

The last of the significant papers on cannabis and schizophrenia published in 2002 (Arseneault *et al.*, 2002) was a short report in the *British Medical Journal*. It was an analysis of data from the Dunedin multidisciplinary health and development study in New Zealand, which had followed 1,037 individuals born in 1972–3 up to the age of 26. Seven hundred and fifty-nine participants were included who were still alive and for whom there were full data available. Information had been collected about psychotic symptoms at the age of 11 and drug use at the ages of 15 and 18, based on self-report. Psychiatric symptoms had been assessed at the age of 26 using a standardised interview schedule that generated Diagnostic and Statistical Manual Fourth Edition (DSM-IV) diagnoses. The purpose of the paper was to test the extent to which the association between cannabis use and schizophrenia was confounded by the use of other recreational drugs. It also explored causality through linking early cannabis use with later schizophrenia, to establish that psychosis did not lead to cannabis use rather than vice versa. The study controlled for gender and parental occupation, using a six-category socio-economic class (SEC) model. The paper makes no mention of controlling for any other factor.

The headline result was that there was a strong association between adolescent cannabis use and schizophrenia aged 26, with a bigger effect in those who first reported cannabis use aged 15. This was taken to reflect an age-related vulnerability or possibly heavier use in those who started taking cannabis younger. Other reported drug use did not affect the findings. When participants who had psychotic symptoms aged 11 were excluded from the analysis, the risk of schizophrenia was still raised, but it was no longer statistically significant. The Odds Ratio for developing schizophrenia was raised (with wide confidence intervals) and statistically significant for cannabis use aged 15, and raised but not statistically significant for cannabis use aged 18. There was an increased risk of schizophrenia at 26 for those who reported psychotic symptoms at 11. The Odds Ratio was higher than for cannabis users, and the level of statistical significance was also higher. There was no association between cannabis use aged 15 and depressive disorder at the age of 26, but there was a statistically significant association between cannabis use at age 18 and later depression.

The real problem with the study is, again, low numbers. Of the 759 participants, 25 had schizophrenia aged 26. The number of individuals who reported cannabis use at 15 and had developed schizophrenia by 26 years was three. Our interpretation of the findings is much the same as it was for the previous two studies. We do not doubt the association. We are far from convinced that confounding factors have been eliminated from the findings, including social deprivation and childhood adversity. We cannot know if the residual effect of these is large enough to account for the findings, but we believe that it is possible.

Those who suggest that the relationship between cannabis use and schizophrenia is causal and that this is now beyond doubt would argue that the association is consistent across studies that use different methodologies and control for confounding factors in different ways. In 2006, a paper was published in the *British Journal of Psychiatry* based on data from a prospective longitudinal study of 152 people with recent onset of first-onset schizophrenia (Barnes *et al.*, 2006). The essential findings were a high rate of substance misuse, with roughly equal numbers misusing alcohol and other substances. Gender and cannabis use had independent effects on age of onset of schizophrenia. However, social factors were not controlled for. The sample was drawn from inner-city West London, but this cannot be taken to mean that the sample was socially homogenous.

It is argued that there is a plausible mechanism connecting schizophrenia and cannabis, as cannabinoid receptors are known to modulate dopamine function. There was a brief period when it seemed that there was a possibility that this area of research might yield a true breakthrough. There seemed to be a link between an environmental factor (cannabis use) and a specific gene polymorphism of known molecular characteristics. The gene in question codes for an enzyme involved in the monoamine systems of the brain.

Like the study reported by Arseneault *et al.* in 2002, this study was based on the Dunedin birth cohort (Caspi *et al.*, 2005). Participants had given blood for DNA analysis as part of their regular contact with the research team. The catechol-O-methyltransferase (COMT) gene has been investigated as a candidate gene in a number of conditions, including schizophrenia. It is located on chromosome 22, which has been implicated in schizophrenia. The COMT gene is an enzyme that is involved in the metabolism of dopamine, which is definitely involved in some way with schizophreniform symptoms. There is a mutation of the COMT gene that substitutes valine for methionine at codon 158, altering the level of biological activity of the enzyme, and thus altering the rate of breakdown of dopamine. The alleles are co-dominant, so that people can have one of three different forms of COMT, with three levels of biological activity: Met/Met, Met/Val and Val/Val. In this study, roughly 50% of subjects were Met/Val, whilst Met/Met and Val/Val were roughly 25% each. The key finding was that early cannabis use was associated with an increased risk of schizophrenia in the Val/Val group and, to a lesser extent the Met/Val group. There was no association between cannabis use and schizophrenia in the Met/Met group.

This was a startling finding. It appeared that the Val substitution conferred a vulnerability to the effects of cannabis, with a greater vulnerability for homozygotes than heterozygotes. As was entirely understandable, the authors of the paper were expansive on the implications of the finding, although it was acknowledged that they required replication. Of course, the study involved exactly the same participants as the previous Dunedin paper on cannabis and schizophrenia, and numbers of people with schizophrenia were low. In 2007, a much larger study was published in the *British Journal of Psychiatry* that contradicted the Dunedin findings (Zammit *et al.*, 2007). Four hundred and ninety-three people with schizophrenia had their COMT polymorphism status assessed, and this was analysed with regard to their history of cannabis use. There was no evidence to support different effects of cannabis use according to COMT polymorphism status. There was no association between schizophrenia, COMT polymorphisms and tobacco use. The possibility of a link between schizophrenia, cannabis and a specific gene polymorphism was no longer credible.

We have not presented a comprehensive review of the literature on cannabis and schizophrenia. There is sufficient here to illustrate the main issues with regard to poverty and genetics. The *Lancet* systematic review in 2007 (Moore *et al.*, 2007) stated:

... pooled analysis revealed an increase in risk of psychosis of about 40% in participants who had ever used cannabis. (page 325)

This is the most widely cited figure. It represents a substantial increase in risk. However, the background population risk of developing schizophrenia is about 1%, so that the personal risk for individual cannabis users of developing schizophrenia is increased by about 0.5%. If we hypothesise that the apparent increase in risk is entirely due to the residual confounding effect of social deprivation, the size of the effect is within the bounds of the plausible. We saw in Chapter 1 that the effect of childhood exposure to severe inner-city deprivation in increasing the risk of developing schizophrenia is considerably greater than 40%. Whilst it is clear that most of the cannabis studies did at least partially control for deprivation, we believe that there is a prima facie case that the measures used were too crude to fully control for it.

Much of the entire literature on schizophrenia and other major mental illnesses uses similarly crude variables to understand and control for social factors. Socio-economic class as measured by occupation or highest level of educational attainment, and urbanicity as defined by city dwelling, supplemented by factors that have an association with social deprivation, such as childhood disturbance and criminality, do partially control for deprivation, but it is unlikely they can completely achieve this. This does not necessarily mean that the studies that use these measures are fatally flawed. In many studies, the rough-and-ready nature of the variables measured does not really matter. Those who feel that a causal relationship between cannabis use and schizophrenia is established are likely to feel that we have taken hold of a few minor and unavoidable flaws in research design and blown them out of proportion. Nonetheless, in our opinion, the causal role of cannabis use is not established, as there are plausible alternative explanations for the findings that have not been adequately explored.

We suggest that the overestimation of the strength of the evidence for a specific causal role for cannabis has had widespread and largely negative consequences. Cannabis users have been criminalised by changes in classification of the drug. A proportion of the population have come to believe that schizophrenia is self-inflicted. Parents worry about the mental health of teenagers whose occasional use of cannabis is unlikely to cause any long-term harm. The major lesson is that it is easy to overestimate the strength of evidence by brushing aside credible alternative explanations for findings, and that the consequences can be unpredictable.

Main points in this chapter

1. A small number of organic brain syndromes are caused by single gene lesions. In the case of Huntington's disease, molecular genetics has advanced knowledge of the disorder considerably.
2. The major mental illnesses are not due to single gene lesions. At present it appears that many different genes have some impact on the risk of developing major mental illness. These genetic risk factors do not seem to be specific to particular diagnoses.
3. Although socio-biology has influential advocates, it is likely that many aspects of human behaviour are not determined by genes and are beyond the influence of natural selection.
4. Although it is widely believed that early cannabis use causes schizophrenia, the association is open to other plausible explanations.
5. Exaggeration of the strength of evidence continues to bedevil psychiatry.

6

Substance misuse

Drug and alcohol use are ubiquitous in the developed countries, and they continue to provoke huge controversy. Harmful substance misuse is a major public health problem, but the supply and use of two of the most damaging substances, alcohol and tobacco, is legal and economically important. Tobacco use is in decline. Whilst overall drug misuse shows little sign of abating, in Western Europe heroin addiction and intravenous drug use show a steady decline (Barrio *et al.*, 2013). Set against this, UK per capita alcohol consumption is at a level that by historical standards is very high.

Does alcohol make you poor?

At the very start of the Industrial Revolution, as modern cities started to form, there was a moral panic over alcohol consumption by the poor. This was the Gin Epidemic of the eighteenth century.[1] There was virtually no control over the production of spirits at the time. Very cheap gin was consumed in large quantities by workers in new urban industries. Public displays of drunkenness were common, and there was particular disquiet about inebriated women. Gin came to be known as Mother's Ruin. There was political concern over the consequences for the economy, public order and morality. Between 1729 and 1751, attempts were made to control production and consumption through a series of Acts of Parliament. These introduced licensing and levies, which were ineffective. Eventually, national gin consumption moderated for other reasons, primarily a sharp rise in price due to conditions in the grain market. The focus of concern was on the poor and on the spread of *moral degeneracy* amongst them. The episode established the main themes in public debate over substance misuse that persist until the present day. This included the belief that drinking caused poverty.

[1] Skinner E (2007) The Gin Craze: Drink, Crime & Women in 18th Century London. *Cultural Shifts* archive.is/http://culturalshifts.com/archives/168 *retrieved 5 April 2013.*

The cause of poverty in developed economies was a key political dispute between the left and the right of mainstream politics until the sudden death of egalitarianism in the 1980s. Until then, the left regarded poverty as an avoidable consequence of a dysfunctional social and economic structure. The right regarded it as a consequence of indolence induced by a counter-productive state safety net of welfare provision, which it was claimed had the effect of undermining desirable values of self-improvement and independence. Without the stultifying effects of welfare provision, these values would encourage the poor to lift themselves from their predicament. In recent decades, the mainstream left has looked to widespread intervention with individuals in order to improve the attitudes and skills of the poor. Recent examples include the national Sure Start scheme (National Evaluation of Sure Start Team, 2010). As mentioned in Chapter 3, the right's position is largely unchanged and the allegedly destructive effects of welfare and social security is the dominant political discourse.

These ideological positions are primarily determined by values associated with conflicting moral stances. Values and morality are irreducible and they do not require evidence to support them. However, if you follow the evidence, it leads to quite different conclusions about the causes of poverty. We do not believe that our perspective is overly coloured by our own values and what we would like to be true. During the Gin Epidemic, it was generally believed that drinking alcohol made people poor, and similar beliefs were articulated by the Temperance Movement in the run-up to US Prohibition in the 1920s. There have been recent proposals to prevent welfare claimants from spending their benefits on alcohol, implicitly reviving this argument. In spite of this, there is no real evidence that alcohol consumption is a major cause of poverty.

In all countries where alcohol is legal there is a group of very heavy drinkers who consume a high proportion of all of the alcohol sold. The lower the total national consumption of alcohol, the higher the proportion that is consumed by heavy drinkers (Babor et al., 2010). In a high-consumption country like the UK, heavy drinkers consume some 30% of all alcohol sold. Clearly in many cases these individuals are prioritising drinking over other imperatives, and this affects their financial well-being. Salience of drinking in people with a serious alcohol problem is so prevalent that it was one of the seven key features of Griffith Edwards' alcohol dependence syndrome (Edwards & Gross, 1976). The fact that drinking can be a cause of individual penury does not automatically imply that drinking is a substantial cause of poverty at a population level.

The relationship between alcohol consumption and social class is not straightforward. Contrary to a popular stereotype, alcohol consumption is not highest amongst the poor. The highest rates of alcohol consumption are amongst the educated middle classes (Office for National Statistics, 2006). Analysis of national consumption figures suggests that higher-income groups consume alcohol more frequently and are more likely to engage in binge drinking than people in lower economic groups (Jefferis et al., 2007; Marmot, 1997). Complete abstinence is commonest in the poorest part of the population. Despite this, poorer people suffer more adverse consequences of the current high levels of alcohol consumption in the UK.

The UK is drowning in alcohol

Over 90 per cent of adults in the UK consume alcohol, and alcoholic beverages are an intrinsic component of British culture. They have a prominent role in social rituals, both casual (such as having a drink with colleagues after work) and formal (such as weddings, christenings and funerals). Alcohol has been regarded as a social problem in Britain intermittently for 2000 years (French, 1884). The unfortunate fact is that excessive consumption of alcohol has toxic effects on every organ system in the body. The boundary between 'safe' and 'harmful' drinking is indistinct. Indeed, in behavioural terms, moderate and heavy consumption are not discrete categories of drinking behaviour, but are on a continuum. It would be foolish to suggest that we could abolish alcohol consumption as a feature of our society. It cannot be completely eliminated, but minimising the harm caused by alcohol is an attainable objective.

Throughout the history of psychiatry, it has been recognised that alcohol consumption complicates and worsens the course and outcome of mental illnesses. Furthermore, drinking has a causal association with some specific disorders. For example, the amnesic syndrome, 'Korsakoff's psychosis', is characterised by profound difficulty in forming new memories. It is most commonly due to thiamine (vitamin B1) deficiency, a nutritional consequence of long-term heavy drinking. The amnesic syndrome can be preceded by acute thiamine deficiency with Wernicke's encephalopathy, or it can have an insidious onset. Alcoholic hallucinosis is a disorder with a characteristic psychopathology (disturbing and vivid auditory hallucinations), course and treatment response, which arises after years of alcohol abuse. It eventually remits with sustained abstinence. Depression is commonly complicated by drinking, which predictably causes mood to deteriorate. In some cases depressive illness can appear to be entirely attributable to alcohol consumption. The mood disorder resolves when the person is persuaded that drinking is part of the problem, not part of the solution, and stops.

The physical ill effects of heavy alcohol consumption are well understood. There are direct causal links between alcohol and liver disease, hypertension, cardiovascular disease, pancreatitis, some cancers and a range of other life-threatening illnesses.

In the light of this, it is uncontroversial to state that alcohol misuse has direct effects, which are biological in nature, in causing and seriously complicating physical and mental illness. Lately, health professionals have become concerned by epidemiological evidence that alcohol-related morbidity and mortality rates are sharply increasing in the UK. The Royal College of Physicians leads a campaigning group, Alcohol Health Alliance UK. In some parts of the country, centrally collected statistics have shown a doubling of alcohol-related deaths in a decade

(Office for National Statistics, 2008). According to the World Health Organization, in the 30 years between 1970 and 2000, deaths from chronic liver disease rose in the UK by over 900% for both men and women (World Health Organization, 2004). Although this is not entirely attributable to increasing alcohol consumption, it is a very significant factor (Leon & Cambridge, 2006).

The increase in alcohol consumption in the UK may not be entirely due to government policy, but this has certainly been a major influence. Although there has been no overt policy to encourage drinking, all administrations between 1979 and 2010 pursued policies that made alcohol more available and more affordable. A progressive reduction in duty relative to price, together with deregulation of retail sale, led to a situation where in the first decade of the twenty-first century alcohol was cheaper and easier to purchase than at any time since 1914, perhaps longer. The inevitable consequence was that per capita consumption steadily increased.

It is hard to accurately quantify the effect of this on the population's mental health, but there is a widespread perception that there has been an increase in the incidence of cerebral disorders where alcohol has a causal role. Cerebral damage related to alcohol misuse is a condition of complex aetiology. Many heavy drinkers are also heavy smokers with poor nutrition, each of which can contribute to the pathological processes affecting the brain. Notwithstanding the difficulties in isolating the effects solely due to alcohol, it appears that presentations of cerebral damage related to drinking are sharply increasing, mainly affecting men in their 50s and 60s who have been drinking to excess for 20 or 30 years (Jauhar & Smith, 2009).

The UK increase in per capita alcohol consumption has been accompanied by significant changes in patterns of alcohol use. In the 1970s, retail sales of alcohol in the UK were heavily regulated. It could only be sold from licensed premises between specified hours. The majority of bars and licensed premises that were accessible to the general public could not sell alcoholic beverages after 11pm. Alcohol for consumption at home was sold from licensed specialist shops ('off-licences') with even shorter opening hours than bars. Generally speaking, beer (representing the largest volume of alcohol sales) was cheaper to consume in public houses than at home. Taxation was much heavier for wines and spirits than for beers.

Pricing structures that encouraged people to drink weaker beverages in bars, and therefore in the company of other people, have subsequently disappeared. Price incentives have reversed, and it is now cheaper to drink at home. Supermarkets routinely sell strong liquor at below cost price as a loss leader. Young people tend to drink spirits before they go out, to avoid purchasing drinks at high cost in pubs and clubs, so that they tend to be intoxicated at the start of a night out rather than just at the end of it. This increases their risk exposure to the inherent dangers associated with intoxication in a public place. Consumption of strong drinks has increased, and brewers have developed cheap super-strength beers and ciders that appear to have the sole purpose of causing intoxication. These are as unpalatable as they are powerful, and they seem to have been developed to satisfy demand in the market from the alcohol-dependent.

There has been a historical pattern whereby women have consumed significantly less alcohol than men. Women are increasing their consumption especially quickly, mainly in the form of wine. Women are more vulnerable to alcohol-related tissue damage compared with men exposed to the same dose. They are catching up with male rates of alcohol-related disease (Office for National Statistics, 2008) as an inevitable consequence of increased consumption. Higher than expected rates of alcohol misuse are now being found amongst older people (St John *et al.*, 2010), although it is not clear whether this is due to an increase in consumption in this age group or due to increased awareness of the problem, with higher rates of diagnosis as a consequence.

The pattern and level of alcohol consumption in the UK is a public health disaster. Even if effective action is taken immediately to reverse the trends, a legacy of death and illness is inevitable for many years to come. The disaster has been facilitated by the avoidable factor of incrementally bad governmental policy decisions. It is tempting to attribute these decisions to collusion between government and alcohol manufacturers. There is certainly evidence of unscrupulousness in the alcohol industry. This is reminiscent of the behaviour of tobacco manufacturers at their worst (Hastings *et al.*, 2010). One might speculate that politicians have encouraged the alcohol epidemic in order to benefit from political support from brewers and increased tax revenues from increases in sales. It is equally likely that policy has been driven by undue faith in the ability of unregulated markets to generate both a thriving economy and social well-being. Policies that are underpinned by ideology often neglect evidence and result in perverse outcomes, even in the absence of malign intention. Governments have been quite willing to take decisive action against smoking, in the face of significant political influence of tobacco manufacturers and adverse tax-revenue consequences.

There is a profound irrationality in the situation. The cost of health care in the UK is mainly met from general taxation. Alcohol is implicated in a high proportion of acute hospital admissions of all types, and chronic illness related to alcohol consumption is expensive to treat. The burden of the cost of treatment of these acute and chronic illnesses falls on an exchequer that has progressively lowered relative taxation of alcohol, with the inevitable consequence of the spread of disease.

Generally speaking, the amount of alcohol-related harm that occurs in a country is directly related to the amount of alcohol consumed, which is powerfully influenced by cost, or at least affordability. The relationship between cost and consumption, and consumption and harm, is relatively fixed. It is not the case that as prices drop, increased consumption is confined to a sub-population with an individual vulnerability to harmful drinking. As national consumption increases, everyone drinks more, recruiting a large number of people from a less harmful to a more harmful level of use. This is reflected in the lower proportion of alcohol use concentrated amongst the heaviest drinkers in high-consumption countries that was mentioned above. This would tend to contradict the Alcoholics Anonymous doctrine that substance dependency is an inherent biological or spiritual vulnerability of individuals. If this was the case, one would expect the increase in consumption to be confined to the vulnerable population, instead of which the whole population is affected and people who would otherwise remain well develop alcohol-related problems.

The determinants of individual drinking behaviour are complex, with a significant contribution from cultural, religious and psychological factors. Nonetheless, it seems clear that a relatively simple and crude structural social factor, namely the cost of alcoholic beverages, has a very large impact at individual and population levels. There is evidence from sophisticated economic modelling that the introduction of a minimum price for a unit of alcohol (10 ml of ethanol) would substantially reduce consumption, especially amongst those groups that are most vulnerable to cheap and nasty super-strength drinks (Booth *et al.*, 2008; Brennan *et al.*, 2008). The UK Government was seriously contemplating implementation of minimum pricing, but, after equivocation and consultation with the alcohol industry, has had a change of heart. The Scottish Parliament has been less timid in committing itself to the policy, but has yet to implement the Alcohol (Minimum Pricing) (Scotland) Act 2012, which is under legal challenge by the Scotch Whisky Association and other representatives of the alcohol industry. Although they claim to be trying to protect consumers from being 'penalised', it is reasonable to infer that manufacturers are concerned because they believe that minimum pricing will reduce sales. Their resistance is an unintended endorsement of the policy.

Alcohol's close relationship with mental illness is an example of the way in which a biological mechanism, namely the toxic effect of ethanol at a cellular level, can be profoundly modulated by social factors. Social factors can affect the dose-related toxicity of alcohol. As described above, alcohol consumption is highest amongst the educated middle class. Despite this, there is an association between alcohol-related death and socio-economic deprivation (Erskine *et al.*, 2010). Rates of admission of poorer people to hospital for problems related to drinking are disproportionately high, despite their relatively low per capita alcohol consumption. This is especially marked for mental and behavioural disorders related to drinking (Deacon *et al.*, 2010; Morleo *et al.*, 2010a).

This phenomenon, whereby exposure to apparently similar illness-provoking factors has a larger effect in poorer parts of the population, is seen in the epidemiology of a number of different conditions. For example, poor smokers are more addicted to cigarettes than wealthier smokers, and the increase in risk of lung cancer for them is greater than a simple extrapolation from smoking prevalence in the two groups would predict (Richardson & Crosier, 2001). This is probably due to the effects of multiple adverse factors that exacerbate the effect of any individual factor. High rates of smoking amongst poorer people, for example, means that cardiovascular disease will tend to combine with the effects of alcohol in causing cerebral damage in this population.

Heavy drinking and smoking are undoubtedly bad lifestyle choices that are sometimes made by people, rich and poor, who are capable of understanding the health implications. The question for anyone who is interested in improving the mental health of the population is whether it is better to try to intervene at an individual level to influence those choices or whether it is better to make structural social interventions that have an impact on the way that people live. At the time of writing, policy makers favour campaigns of health education to reduce 'irresponsible' drinking, some aimed at the whole population, some targeting sections of the population where drinking is seen to be particularly problematic, such as the young. It is not the case that these campaigns fail to influence individual behaviour. However, they do not have a sufficiently large and continuous effect to overcome the influence of powerful structural incentives to drink, such as affordability (Bailey *et al.*, 2011). Furthermore, these campaigns are predicated on the belief that drinking behaviour dichotomises into 'safe', 'responsible' drinking and 'harmful', 'irresponsible' drinking. Drinking behaviour is continuously distributed, with no neat boundary between the safe and the harmful, so that targeting harmful drinking, even if it were effective, can only ever have an effect on part of the problem.

The population's behaviour with regard to smoking illustrates the limited impact of health education, at least in the short term. As soon as convincing findings emerged on the health consequences of smoking, the medical profession radically changed their behaviour, and rates of smoking amongst doctors rapidly reduced (Doll *et al.*, 1994). Most of the rest of the population were much slower to change. In the face of incontrovertible evidence of the dangers of smoking, rates of smoking were initially static or possibly actually increased amongst some parts of the population, such as young women in the lowest socio-economic classes (Bostock, 2003). There was then an overall decrease, and smoking slowly became less socially acceptable, but the changes occurred over 50 years, and many people died prematurely in the meantime. The more recent ban on smoking in enclosed public spaces appears to have had a profound effect on attitudes to the habit. The ban is widely accepted and adhered to, it has reduced rates of smoking (Bauld, 2011) and it has made smoking in work and social settings profoundly unacceptable. Although it may be argued that the prior process of health education was necessary to achieve acceptance and adherence to the ban, nonetheless the effectiveness of this single, simple social structural intervention stands in stark contrast to the limited effects of prior health awareness campaigns. The only other intervention that has had a comparable effect on smoking has been progressive increases in price, which is another structural intervention (Reed, 2009).

Mortality, smoking and severe mental illness

It has been known for a long time that people with severe mental illness are at risk of dying young. Schizophrenia, bipolar affective disorder and delusional disorder are all associated with suicide, but there is also a substantial risk of premature death from physical disease. People with severe mental illness are roughly twice as likely to smoke as the rest of the population. They are more likely to live in deprived areas and to take medication that has adverse metabolic effects. This creates a challenge in understanding the epidemiology of premature death and it has been difficult to tease out the various factors in order to understand the nature of the increased risk.

Alongside the general recognition of raised mortality rates, there has been some ambiguity as to which diseases contribute to this. Some studies have suggested that an increased mortality due to some causes is offset by a lower mortality due to others. This follows findings of a lower than expected rate of some cancers, with the suggestion that this might be a consequence of a putative protective effect of a number of medications (Grinshpoon et al., 2005). A very large British cohort study (Osborn et al., 2007) of people with severe mental illness (i.e. psychosis) confirmed that overall mortality rates were raised and did not find any reduced mortality due to cancers. The increased risk was found to be due mainly to cardiovascular disease and lung cancer. After adjustment for the effects of antipsychotic medication, smoking and social deprivation, mortality was still higher than expected. The authors concluded that increased mortality associated with severe mental illness was not wholly explained by these factors. However, whilst medication and smoking had been assessed at the individual level, social deprivation was assessed by the level of deprivation in the neighbourhood of the general practice where the person was registered. As the degree of deprivation can vary considerably between individuals residing in a particular area, it is possible that this variable was not adequately controlled for in the analysis. It is unclear whether the remaining excess mortality was related to mental illness, social deprivation or some other factor.

A number of hypotheses have been offered to explain the elevated rates of smoking amongst people with mental illness. Smoking is common in institutions where there is little fruitful activity, and institutionalism was a plausible explanation when mental health care was mainly delivered in large mental hospitals. However, these institutions closed long ago and there is still an excess of smokers amongst people with mental illness. It has been suggested that smoking represents an attempt to self-medicate using nicotine to influence mood, but there is no real evidence that smoking has a positive effect on mood. Alternatively, it has been suggested that smoking might reduce some of the adverse effects of medication. Smoking causes enzyme induction and reduces blood levels of some antipsychotics. It makes people feel more alert, which might counter a 'drugged' feeling. Some studies have shown raised rates of smoking before the onset of mental illness, leading to the suggestion that smoking might cause mental illness (Lasser et al., 2000).

It seems something of a coincidence that rates of smoking in the lowest social classes are twice the rate for the general population (Marmot, 1997). This is a very similar difference to that seen in people with serious mental illness, who are disproportionately drawn from these social classes. Indeed, Graham has described being a smoker as 'a social marker of class-related disadvantage' (Graham, 2012, page 91). Smoking is prevalent amongst the marginalised and the stigmatised, and it has been suggested that smoking control programmes have unintentionally not only made smoking unacceptable, they have also made smokers unacceptable. Smoking is perceived as blameworthy, an anti-social and self-inflicted assault on health. The social status of marginalised smokers subsumes other categories that are beyond the person's control such as social class or mental illness.

Notwithstanding this example of coming to see people with problems as people who are a problem, there have been concerted efforts to tackle high mortality rates through interventions aimed at smoking. There is no evidence that people with mental illness are any less likely to quit in smoking cessation programmes than anybody else (Prochaska, 2011). However, much of the debate has centred on whether people admitted to psychiatric inpatient facilities should be prevented from smoking. The argument has been that it is wrong to admit people to hospital and then to collude with a behaviour that is destructive to health. It is also argued that admission to hospital represents an opportunity to intervene in a group at high risk of premature death from smoking. Prochaska refutes a number of spurious arguments against making psychiatric inpatient units completely smoke-free. What she doesn't deal with is the question of human rights. Freedom isn't meaningful if it excludes the right to make bad decisions. If someone is detained in hospital, is it right to prevent an activity that is lawful and neutral with regard to recovery from the condition that led to their detention in the first instance? How can a paternalistic intervention at this point be consistent with a Recovery model (see Chapter 9)?

Drugs

Drug use in the UK is common across all social classes. There is controversy as to how harmful this might be compared to the use of legal substances such as tobacco and alcohol (Nutt *et al.*, 2010). Recreational drug use is now an intrinsic element of the social life of young people and, to a lesser extent, a proportion of older people too. Patterns of drug use change, and new substances become available. To the older observer, some fashions in drug use can be puzzling, such as the current widespread recreational use of anaesthetic agents such as ketamine and nitrous oxide. It would be wrong to characterise this type of drug use as harmless. Quite apart from adverse effects on users, widespread use of illicit drugs channels very large sums of money into organised crime. However, the majority of users outgrow drug use unscathed, and even senior politicians in the USA and UK acknowledge youthful dalliances with drugs.

In contrast to the non-dependent use of stimulants, hallucinogens and cannabis, the use of heroin is strongly associated with social deprivation, social marginalisation and criminality (Seddon, 2006). To a large extent crack cocaine use follows similar patterns to heroin. Policy makers have tended to construe heroin use as a kind of contagion that draws people into criminality. There is little doubt that this can happen. Nonetheless, there is clear evidence that criminality is often well established before people start taking heroin, and even some suggestion of reverse causality. Criminality might cause heroin dependency by placing people in social environments where heroin use is accepted. Criminality involves a mind set that seeks short-term benefits and ignores long-term consequences. In a significant proportion of people, drug use and criminality probably have origins in attitudes and social environments that promote both behaviours. It is not the case that exposure to opiates necessarily leads to dependency. There is good evidence that controlled use is common (Warburton *et al.*, 2005), which is not to deny that heroin is highly destructive in the lives of a proportion of people who use it.

People who are heroin-dependent are highly likely to have multiple disadvantages in their background. They are likely to have problems with unstable housing and homelessness, long-term unemployment and recurrent imprisonment. The price of heroin has dropped owing to market saturation and it has become more affordable. Nonetheless, men who use heroin are often involved in acquisitive crime and women are often involved in sex work. Here is a constellation of disadvantage writ large (see Chapter 3). It is highly unlikely that people in this situation would be leading lives in the mainstream of society if one could magically abolish the street heroin supply. Furthermore, some people living on the margins of society find benefits in belonging to heroin-using sub-cultures. The psychological barriers to initiation into opiate use may be weaker for people who see little reason to be optimistic about the future and who feel that they have little to lose. Opiate addicts form inward-looking social networks with places to go and things to do that are entirely separate from mainstream life (although they co-exist alongside each other). This can be attractive to people struggling with barren, hopeless, unsatisfying lives. People do not necessarily choose drug addiction in the spirit of reckless self-destruction. The benefits are real if a comfortable 'normal' life seems unattainable.

Addiction is a moral concept

There has been serious concern for some time in the USA over dependency on opioid analgesics (Compton & Volkow, 2006). In 2008, more Americans died of overdose of opioid analgesics than died from overdosage of heroin and cocaine (Warner *et al.*, 2011). The problem has been little researched in the UK, but there is good reason to suppose that there are similar problems here. UK opioid prescriptions in primary care are rising rapidly. Within the literature from pain management clinics, opioid analgesic misuse is seen predominantly as a consequence of people with established drug dependency misconstruing themselves as suffering from chronic pain in order to secure prescribed opioids. There is little published about iatrogenic dependence or about dependence as a consequence of treatment of bona fide chronic pain (categories that overlap but are not identical). Clinicians have the impression that both problems are common.

It has been difficult to settle on a definition of addiction that enjoys general support within health services and the research community. The everyday understanding of the concept of *addiction* bleeds into clinical practice. The term is a form of professional vernacular rather than an internally consistent scientific concept.

There are contradictions within the concept as it is used, for example, in understanding *addiction* as an illness but one that comes about through choices and intentions. In other words, it is usually understood that *addiction* is a volitional phenomenon, which means that there is a moral element to the problem. *Addiction* has a shameful connotation. Consequently, professionals attempt to eliminate *addicts* from services intended for the blameless, and the blameless are defined as not being *addicted* even when they cannot control their use of dependency-forming prescription drugs. Drugs such as antidepressants that do not cause a pleasurable intoxication are defined as non-addictive, notwithstanding the fact that some people get withdrawal symptoms when they try to stop using them (which is labelled a 'discontinuation syndrome').

In this vernacular use of the concept of *addiction*, those who use drugs therapeutically and those who are addicted are distinguished from each other by the intentions they had when they commenced taking the drug. The degree of blame attached to drug use is diminished where the street addict is seen as self-medicating, for example, if they have a prior mental illness. Hence *inadvertent addiction* appears to be an oxymoron, because intention is part of the de facto meaning of *addiction*.

It can be difficult to get practitioners to see that the common feature of dysfunctional substance use is the inability to stop despite adverse consequences. This means that people with chronic pain whose drug use has become dysfunctional run two risks. Complaining of continuing pain, they may be regarded by physicians as in need of more drugs, when what would be helpful to them is to take less medication. There is an equal and paradoxical risk that they press their case for more medication too hard and physicians come to see them as addicted, and therefore *necessarily* not in pain or not likely to benefit from treatment of pain at all.

Substance-misuse practitioners will no doubt object to understanding professional responses to substance misuse as a moral reaction on the grounds that the moral model of addiction is outmoded and discredited. This is true, but the ideas linger on. Concepts of addiction have deep roots in religious thinking (Cook, 2009). Alcoholics Anonymous and the Minnesota Method are highly influential. They explicitly place spirituality and faith at the heart of their model of addiction and recovery. There is a reluctance to regard iatrogenic drug dependence as a phenomenon comparable to alcoholism or street drug addiction. An objection may be raised that street drug users are demographically and clinically distinct from people with chronic pain who cannot stop over-use of opioids, but this reasoning is tautological. If street heroin users are defined as 'proper' addicts then other groups with difficulties relating to substance use will always fall outside of the definition of addiction. It is hard to find anything that distinguishes iatrogenic and street addicts with respect to the actual dysfunctional use of a drug. Tolerance, withdrawal symptoms, craving and inability to function owing to the effects of intoxication all occur in both groups. It appears that there is a reluctance to classify the iatrogenic addict with the street addict because the latter are social pariahs. They are perceived to be poor, socially chaotic people who have little in common with honest citizens whose drug use is therapeutically sanctioned. The distinction between them is a moral judgement. Indeed, even the word 'iatrogenic' emphasises that the blame lies elsewhere, not with the person themself. One could debate at some length as to whether addiction really does involve choices or not, but it is quite certain that regarding it as a blameworthy choice is seriously unhelpful in trying to assist people to become drug-free.

There is a literature that explores the nature or essence of addiction. Some would expand the concept to include gambling addiction or sex addiction. Others would regard these as entirely different behaviours to substance dependence, or consider the application of an addiction model to them as an inappropriate reframing of self-indulgent excess. Leaving aside the merits of these arguments, what is striking is that the concept of addiction is only ever applied to behaviour that is regarded as undesirable, which would tend to underline the moral origins of the concept.

It is sometimes suggested that the essential features of addiction to substances are tolerance (the drug has less effect on extended exposure), withdrawal (there is a specific withdrawal syndrome that is seen on discontinuation) and craving (a subjective compulsion to seek out and use the drug). It has long been accepted that benzodiazepines are addictive, as all three features are seen. Although they are prescription medications, they are also widely traded and used as street drugs. The argument that selective serotonin reuptake inhibitor antidepressants (SSRIs) are not addictive has rested on the fact that, whilst there is a discontinuation syndrome, tolerance and craving are not seen. It is difficult to see what difference this makes to a person who struggles to stop taking SSRIs. They might reasonably conclude that they are suffering from an iatrogenic addiction. Quite apart from the inconvenience of regarding these valuable therapeutic agents as addictive, there is another argument against regarding them as addictive. Unlike benzodiazepines, hardly anyone finds SSRI use pleasurable. This is yet another example of the implicit moral dimension to the concept of addiction.

There are other problems with the concept of addiction. If you are taking a substance like an opioid analgesic that unequivocally causes physical dependence, but you never try to either increase the dose or discontinue the medication, can you be regarded as addicted to it? If not, when you do eventually try to stop and you suffer withdrawals and craving, are you now addicted? Did the addiction start when you tried to stop or were you addicted all along?

The concept of dysfunctional drug use (the person cannot discontinue drug use at will despite adverse consequences) avoids these difficulties, but it is not commonly recognised or accepted. People with an addiction are stigmatised, marginalised and regarded as blameworthy. Even substance misuse services demand that addicts should show a particular form of contrition known as motivation in order to receive or benefit from treatment.

Many people who misuse substances find themselves in a difficult position with respect to securing care or treatment for their problems as they are regarded by services as The Wrong Kind of Patient. This is a widespread phenomenon which affects people beyond those with dysfunctional drug use.

The Wrong Kind of Patient

When health professionals working in services of any type, physical or psychiatric, are asked about the problems they face in their work, they almost invariably say that they spend too much time treating the Wrong Kind of Patient. They have special expertise in treating particular problems, but too many of the patients they actually see have other complicating problems that frustrate their efforts to deploy their skills properly. The service has criteria and care pathways, but complicating factors cut across them. The patients tend to be too old; or they have too many secondary diagnoses; or they have attitudes and lifestyles that inhibit treatment adherence and change; or they take alcohol and drugs and this tends to neutralise the benefits of treatment. The NHS spends most of its time treating the Wrong Kind of Patient. Illness does not strike at random, it disproportionately affects those with multiple problems, caught in constellations of disadvantage. Most patients have complicated, atypical illnesses and are therefore at risk of being deemed the Wrong Kind of Patient. It is enough to make you wonder if we have the Wrong Kind of Health Service. We return to this theme later.

One really damaging aspect of being regarded as the Wrong Kind of Patient is that health professionals often see you as being responsible for your own ill health and resent having to treat you at all. For example, the highly questionable but seemingly indestructible concept of drug-induced psychosis provides a conceptual framework that leads to the exclusion of one type of Wrong Kind of Patient from services.

Drug-induced psychosis

Although it has long been known that intoxication with some substances can induce very strange mental states, the modern concept of drug-induced psychosis originates in Phillip Connell's seminal work in the 1950s on amphetamine psychosis (Connell, 1958). Connell showed that intoxication with amphetamine could provoke a transient state with psychopathology identical to paranoid schizophrenia, that this was relatively common at the time, and that symptoms were related to the presence of amphetamine in the body. From around the same time, Sam Cohen, later Professor of Psychiatry at the London Hospital Medical College, started publishing papers suggesting that a significant proportion of people who presented to services as psychotic were suffering from the effects of alcohol or drug abuse. He suggested that it was inappropriate to treat them as if they had a functional psychosis such as schizophrenia. Cohen continued to publish in this vein until the end of his career. For example, he claimed that drug-induced psychosis was extremely common, accounting for up to a half of all admissions for psychosis at his hospital in 1985 (Cohen & Johnson, 1988). He stated that this mainly affected women, and drew attention to his belief that in many cases of drug-induced psychosis, there was no biochemical evidence of alcohol or drug

Box 2 Classification of potential relationships between psychosis and substance use

- Intoxication mimicking functional psychosis *e.g. amphetamine psychosis*
- Pathoplastic reactions in functional psychosis *e.g. cannabis intoxication in mania leading to schizophreniform symptoms*
- Chronic hallucinosis induced by substance abuse *e.g. alcoholic hallucinosis, LSD flashbacks*
- Drug-induced relapse of functional psychosis
- Withdrawal states *e.g. Delirium Tremens*
- Other reactions:
  - ○ intoxication with clouding of consciousness *e.g. opiates*
  - ○ post-intoxication depression *e.g. post-cocaine crash*
  - ○ panic attacks
- True drug-induced psychosis *e.g. chronic psychosis following stimulant use. Symptoms start with drug use but persist beyond intoxication. Validity doubtful and syndrome may not exist*
- Early drug use causing later functional psychosis *e.g. cannabis and schizophrenia*

use, in other words that the psychosis could persist after the elimination of the drug. In the 1990s he continued to take the view that people suffering from drug-induced psychosis should be held responsible for their actions, that they should be advised, and if necessary supported, to discontinue substance misuse, but that they should not be offered treatment for psychosis as if they had a mental illness (Cohen, 1996).

Deconstructing drug-induced psychosis

Others took a different view. A classification of states that fall under the rubric 'drug-induced psychosis' was proposed, suggesting an alternative and more meaningful terminology (Poole & Brabbins, 1996) (see Box 2). The classification has never been seriously criticised and remains valid. The paper further suggested that where people have psychotic symptoms the treatment should generally be the same irrespective of causation. This proved controversial. Amongst those who resisted this approach were some very eminent psychiatrists who went so far as to say that as a consequence of the alleged conflation of drug-induced psychosis and schizophrenia *'Schizophrenia may be getting a bad name undeservedly'* (Davidson & Roth, 1996, page 651). The desire to separate the blameless who are diagnosed with mental illness from the culpable who have brought their condition on themselves through drug taking could not be clearer.

It can be seen from Box 2 that the possibility of a causal role of cannabis was not dismissed. It was suggested that true drug-induced psychosis should logically be defined as a psychosis commencing with drug use, persisting beyond the elimination of the drug from the body and having features to distinguish it from other types of psychosis such as schizophrenia. It should be noted that there was scepticism that such a state actually existed.

The point was that, in keeping with Davidson and Roth's comments, drug-induced psychosis tended to be diagnosed where the patient was aggressive or frequently relapsed or displayed other undesirable features. Some clinicians felt that the diagnosis of drug-induced psychosis was used to exclude from services people with schizophrenia who happened to have taken drugs, and that sometimes the use of drugs was an inference that was made to explain the patient's failure to get better or to do as they were told. Since 30% to 50% of people with schizophrenia and bipolar affective disorder misuse drugs or alcohol, there appeared to be a good chance that causality was the other way round and that psychosis was inducing drug (or alcohol) use.

Contemporary studies of drug-induced psychosis

Efforts to eliminate the use of *drug-induced psychosis* as a routine diagnosis failed. The concept is alive and well. In 2004, there was a systematic review of the extensive literature on stimulant psychosis (Curran *et al.*, 2004), much of it originating in Japan where a persistent stimulant psychosis was believed to be common. The findings were congruent with the classification published eight years earlier. There was very limited evidence for a kindling effect of stimulants, analogous to epilepsy, where symptoms are provoked at progressively decreased thresholds. Although there is a tendency to assume the existence of a chronic stimulant psychosis, recent papers continue to acknowledge ambiguities over the relationship with schizophrenia per se (e.g. Lichlyter *et al.*, 2011).

There have been studies following the course of mental illness in people diagnosed with drug-induced psychosis. For example, an interesting study from Demark was published in 2005 (Arendt *et al.*, 2005) that used data from the Danish Psychiatric Central Register to follow up 535 patients who were diagnosed with cannabis-induced psychosis on their first contact with psychiatric services. Follow-up was for at least three years. They were compared with people who presented with first-episode schizophrenia spectrum disorder and no history of cannabis use. Almost half of the cannabis-induced psychosis patients went on to be diagnosed with schizophrenia spectrum disorder. The cannabis cases had an earlier age of onset of schizophrenia spectrum disorder than the non-cannabis cases. The authors did briefly discuss alternative explanations for the findings, including the fact that they had not collected information regarding socio-economic status. However, they firmly concluded '*our study shows that cannabis induced psychotic symptoms are an important risk factor for subsequent development of severe psychopathological disorder*'. Many of the cannabis patients were treated as outpatients initially, and the length of admission for those with cannabis-induced psychosis was shorter that those with schizophrenia spectrum disorder. Subsequent studies including all drug-induced psychoses, not just those involving cannabis, from the UK (Komuravelli *et al.*, 2011) and from Finland (Niemi-Pynttäri *et al.*, 2013) have shown high rates of change of diagnosis to schizophrenia on follow-up. Both Scandinavian studies were large record linkage studies, and the authors emphasised that drug-induced psychosis is a precursor to schizophrenia. Only the UK authors of the smaller clinical study took the view that the participants might have had schizophrenia all along and that the inference of a causal role for substance misuse was likely to have been incorrect.

The concept lingers on

It is impossible to be certain whether there is such a thing as a true drug-induced psychosis. It might appear that the debate is about research methods and scientific rigour. However, there is no doubt that people who use drugs or alcohol and who experience psychosis have difficulty in securing good-quality services (Evans-Lacko & Thornicroft, 2010). Drug-induced psychosis, dual diagnosis and cannabis use causing later psychosis (which could appropriately be labelled *tardive psychosis*) refer to rather different phenomena. They are routinely conflated in the literature. It is not surprising to find that policy makers, the media, the general public and many psychiatrists believe that it is well established that drug use, especially use of cannabis, causes life-long mental illness. Leaving aside the scientific issues, there are at least two prominent adverse consequences of this hypothesis being treated as a fact.

Firstly, patients and families often believe that schizophrenia has been caused by cannabis use, with a good deal of recrimination and self-reproach as a consequence. Although it is important to try to help people with mental illness to discontinue cannabis use (because irrespective of a putative causal role, taking cannabis is seriously problematic when people have a major mental illness), a burden of guilt or blame is unhelpful.

Secondly, as discussed in Chapter 5, there has been a huge media furore about cannabis causing schizophrenia. As is its wont, the British tabloid press has disregarded facts and wildly exaggerated the risks of cannabis use, irrespective of fine-grain arguments about causality. The press are quite capable of doing this without assistance, but some researchers have energetically briefed the media and politicians about a causal role. This has contributed to utter confusion in UK drugs policy. In 2009, the Advisory Council on the Misuse of Drugs (ACMD) reviewed the evidence on cannabis and 3,4-methylenedioxymethamphetamine (Ecstasy; MDMA). A few years earlier cannabis had been legally downgraded, and penalties for possession had been reduced. The law was being disregarded by users and much of the criminal justice system in any case. Reclassification coincided with a reduction in use, though this may have occurred independently of the change in the law. The ACMD recommended down-classification of MDMA. The Home Secretary, Jacqui Smith, over-ruled her own scientific advisers, citing contrary advice from eminent researchers. Cannabis was up-graded and MDMA was not reclassified. The chairman of ACMD, Professor David Nutt, continued to publically state that alcohol and tobacco were more dangerous than MDMA and cannabis, which was an interpretation of the evidence that was difficult to fault. He stated that the classification of drugs should follow the current scientific evidence, which was what the law was supposed to achieve. As a direct consequence of making these statements in the public domain, Nutt was sacked by Smith's successor as Home Secretary, Alan Johnson.

The problem with reclassification is that it is known that drug classification has no impact on the decisions that people make about whether to use drugs or not. If the reclassification of cannabis was intended to protect users, it failed. The only tangible result was that users were more likely to be sent to prison if they were caught in possession of cannabis by the police. Far from protecting people with mental health problems who used cannabis, imprisonment was likely to worsen their practical problems. Even researchers who strongly believed that cannabis use causes schizophrenia acknowledged that increasing criminal penalties was a perverse and unintended outcome.

Even if cannabis does not cause schizophrenia, it remains a bad thing for teenagers to do regularly, with a wide range of well-established adverse effects. Cannabis use is bad for people with major mental illness. It can provoke aggression by inducing irritability. The possibility that there is a small increase in risk to individual cannabis smokers of developing schizophrenia is not the most pressing concern about the drug. The recognition that cannabis cannot be eradicated completely and effective measures to reduce harm related to its use would be helpful to a large number of people who suffer ill effects.

Aggressive prohibition, based on the suggestion that it would be possible to prevent hundreds of cases of schizophrenia if cannabis were completely eliminated from the UK, is only a reasonable policy recommendation for a scientist to make if it is true and if it is achievable. No country in the world can claim to have eliminated cannabis use. There are no measures presently under consideration that have any significant chance of achieving this. Lobbying by researchers and journalists led to an increase in penalties for cannabis possession. The ostensible point of the exercise was to protect users, instead of which criminal justice sanctions were applied to them. The entire story is a salutary lesson for clinical researchers who stray into the political arena.

Main points in this chapter

1. Whilst the use of tobacco and intravenous drugs is abating, UK alcohol consumption is extremely high.
2. Poorer people have relatively modest per capita levels of alcohol consumption but suffer disproportionately high levels of alcohol-related harm.

3. People with serious mental illness have raised mortality rates. In part this is due to high rates of substance misuse (especially smoking), poor nutrition and social deprivation.

4. Heroin use has a strong association with severe deprivation and disadvantage. Causality in the link between heroin and crime may run in either direction.

5. Concepts of substance misuse and addiction have an implicit moral dimension that is disapproving and condemnatory.

6. 'Dual diagnosis' and 'drug-induced psychosis' are just two of the labels that are given by services to the people they least like treating and who they regard as the Wrong Kind of Patients.

7

Mechanisms

The present state of knowledge about the relationship between mental ill health and poverty, set out in previous chapters, allows us to make a number of general statements with some confidence. Poverty is associated with physical and mental ill health. As far as one can tell, it seems that causality primarily runs from poverty to mental illness. Whilst having a mental illness has a range of adverse social consequences, poverty is a powerful risk factor for developing mental illness in the first place. Growing up and living in deprived inner-city areas is associated with a particularly increased risk of developing schizophrenia in adulthood. Poverty is by no means the only social factor that has an impact on the risk of developing a mental illness. For example, in some ethnic groups in the UK, parental or grandparental migration has an independent effect on the risk of developing schizophrenia.

These effects do not seem to be a simple reflection of exposure to non-specific social stress. What mechanism or mechanisms might account for these observations? Is it likely that poverty is a causal factor in itself, or is it more likely that the impact of poverty is mediated by psychological or physical factors that have pathophysiological or psychopathological consequences which manifest themselves as mental illness?

There have been extensive efforts to identify specific non-hereditary risk factors for various disorders, particularly schizophrenia. Candidates have included developmental mechanisms (for example, childhood adversity including childhood sexual abuse), psychological mechanisms (for example, social defeat), neurological disadvantage caused by obstetric adversity or infectious agents (such as toxoplasmosis), and exposure to environmental toxins (for example, air pollution). These mechanisms are not necessarily mutually exclusive.

Childhood adversity

Whole populations of children are exposed to some types of adversity, such as low income. Many people are exposed to individual childhood adversity in the form of abuse or neglect. This can include physical, sexual and emotional abuse. There is evidence that exposure to childhood sexual abuse may have a specific relationship with psychotic symptoms in adulthood. Much of the research exploring this relationship has been conducted within an experimental psychology framework. Research psychologists tend to be sceptical of the validity of syndromic diagnosis in mental disorders. They are more interested in the mechanisms that might connect adversity and trauma to specific symptoms or psychological experiences.

In studies of the general population from across the world, a very high proportion of people (perhaps as many as a third of women) report at least one unwelcome sexual experience before the age of 16 years (e.g. Briere & Elliott, 2003; Barth et al., 2012). Such experiences range from being a victim of exhibitionism to being a victim of rape. The severity of these experiences and the distress caused by them varies. Figures are somewhat lower for the type of abuse that is most developmentally damaging. Nonetheless, the proportion of the population exposed to this form of childhood adversity is shockingly high. Across the full range of psychiatric diagnoses, from personality disorder to psychosis, reports by patients of childhood abuse are higher than the rate amongst the general population (Read et al., 2003).

A meta-analysis (Varese et al., 2012) has examined the associations between childhood adversity, trauma and psychosis. The childhood adversity reported included sexual abuse, physical abuse, emotional or psychological abuse, neglect, parental death, and bullying. For all types of childhood adversity the Odds Ratio for adult mental illness was 2.78. In other words, people with psychosis were much more likely to have been exposed to childhood adversity of these types than controls. The Odds Ratio was similar when three different types of study were analysed alone: patient–control studies (OR = 2.72); epidemiological cross-sectional studies (OR = 2.99); and prospective studies (OR = 2.75). In this meta-analysis, no specific trauma emerged as a stronger predictor of psychosis than any other. The adverse effect of physical abuse was as great as the effect of sexual abuse.

Cumulative effects of childhood adversity

Other evidence has suggested that there is a dose response to childhood adversity. In other words the risk of adult psychosis becomes progressively greater with increasing exposure to adversity during childhood. Shevlin and colleagues (Shevlin et al., 2007a) showed that there is a cumulative effect from different types of abuse. People experiencing one type of childhood abuse had an Odds Ratio of 2.12 for the risk of developing psychosis; for two types, the Odds Ratio was 3.89; and for three or more, the Odds Ratio was 7.89. This study also showed that males who were raped as children showed a larger increase in risk of adult psychosis than females who had similar childhood experiences.

Whilst there is no consistent pattern linking any particular form of abuse with specific diagnoses, the picture with regard to childhood abuse and specific psychotic symptoms is different. A recent study using data from a community survey (Bentall *et al.*, 2012) has confirmed previous findings that there is an association between disrupted early-attachment relationships (in the form of institutional care) and adult paranoid symptoms. There is a separate association between childhood sexual abuse, especially rape, and auditory hallucinations. This study showed a 'dose response' relationship.

Findings of such studies are fairly consistent, and are largely the same amongst people who have a diagnosis of bipolar affective disorder as those diagnosed with schizophrenia (Hammersley *et al.*, 2003). It is known that a large proportion of the population suffer from experiences, such as hearing voices, that appear to be similar to psychotic phenomena. The relationship between pseudo-psychotic experiences, which resemble psychosis but are qualitatively different, mild psychotic symptoms, which differ from psychosis only in severity, and full-blown psychosis is far from clear. For example, there are findings (Shevlin *et al.*, 2007b) showing a specific relationship between childhood sexual abuse and visual hallucinations, with only childhood rape and molestation showing a significant association with auditory hallucinations. Tactile hallucinations were associated with physical abuse, rape and molestation in childhood. There was a cumulative effect. However, neither visual nor tactile hallucinations are common or prominent clinical symptoms of psychosis. Although a high degree of specificity between trauma and the form of symptoms can make sense in terms of tentative psychological mechanisms, it makes less sense in the face of the fact that the most prominent symptoms of psychosis are thought disorder, disorganisation and fear. This does not discredit the findings. It does pose questions about the meaning of the findings for syndromal psychosis.

Childhood adversity as a cause of psychosis

A great deal of evidence on childhood adversity and psychosis has accumulated over the past 15 years. It appears that one of the reasons that the association between childhood experience and psychosis has been overlooked is that clinicians are reluctant to ask patients with psychotic symptoms about childhood abuse (Read & Fraser, 1998). Presumably clinicians do not press this line of inquiry on the assumption that where the patient is psychotic such a history does not matter, or perhaps because they fear that the subject may be disturbing for the patient to discuss, with a risk of worsening their mental state. There are a number of models for the psychological mechanisms mediating between childhood adversity and adult symptoms, but at present these can only be speculative.

'Traumagenic' neuro-developmental models have been devised on the basis of these findings. These models are seductive in their effort to unite the psychological, social and biological threads in the understanding of psychosis. The problem is that it is difficult to find hard evidence in support of them. The models offered so far are too unsophisticated to be convincing to the uncommitted observer.

There have been a series of criticisms suggesting that the findings with regard to childhood adversity do not necessarily demonstrate a causal flow from abuse to psychosis. There have been suggestions that the childhood prodromal manifestations of schizophrenia might place children at increased risk of abuse. Whilst such manifestations are known to exist in a proportion of children who go on to develop psychosis (see below), this is a weak and inadequate explanation. There have been suggestions that recollections of childhood abuse are based on adult symptomatology; in other words that they are a retrospective form of paranoia. This is contradicted by a number of studies which strongly suggest that people who report child adversity are accurate in their recollections (Fisher et al., 2011a) and that people with psychosis are as accurate in their reporting of childhood trauma as people without psychosis (Goodman et al., 1997; Fisher et al., 2011b). Such accounts do not alter when people recover from mental illness.

A more salient argument is that childhood trauma and adversity does not arise in discrete dose packages, but as part of constellations of disadvantage (see Chapter 3), and that certain types of abuse may be markers of high levels of generally poor childhood experience and low levels of parental care and protection. It seems that incest is more damaging than sexual abuse by non-kin (Read & Argylle, 1999), which illustrates that the effect of violations, even when severe, has an important contextual element. Childhood adversity has a strong association with later adult adversity, which might confound the association. Abuse of adults is more difficult to reliably identify than abuse of children. Any sexual contact with a child is intrinsically abusive. An adult pattern of recurrent abusive relationships involves value judgements that can be difficult to operationalise, particularly when the abuse is emotional rather than physical.

The evidence on childhood adversity lends strong support to the pivotal role of psychosocial factors in the genesis of serious mental illness. The link with the evidence on poverty is imperfect. It cannot be assumed that the high risk of people who grow up in difficult socio-economic conditions is mediated by a high risk of parental failure and abuse. Indeed, such an assumption would tend to illustrate the stigma of poverty in modern UK society rather than a robust scientific model.

Childhood adversity certainly has an immediate impact on people during childhood. Children looked after by local authorities suffer high levels of mental health difficulties (Ford et al., 2007). Compared with other children they suffer high rates of all types of psychopathology and developmental problems. This is true after controlling for educational and physical factors. Rates are higher for children looked after in residential settings rather than in foster care.

Social defeat

Social defeat is a putative psychosocial mechanism suggested as the mediating factor between deprived urban childhood and adult schizophrenia (Selten & Cantor-Graee, 2007). There is a prima facie appeal to the idea that a difficult childhood instils a belief in children that they have little control over their own lives. As suggested in Chapter 1, they have their faces pressed up against the shop window of life without ever being able to enter. It is not difficult to see that this might have specific consequences for the way that interpersonal experience is processed in adulthood, or that the continual stress of social defeat might have an impact on endocrine, immunological and neurotransmitter systems. The potential explanatory power of the concept is not clearly reflected in the available evidence. There is some conceptual confusion over the nature of social defeat, which contains a degree of tautology; deprived children become deprived adults who feel deprived.

Luhrmann (2007) defines social defeat as an actual social encounter in which one person physically or symbolically loses to another. According to him, the encounter is contested, or experienced as contested, and the individual has the experience of losing. According to Luhrmann, social defeat is not equivalent to helplessness, demoralisation or anomie. In this model, social defeat is a transient state that arises repetitively ('[...] the daily experience of survival with serious psychotic illness is one of repeated social failure'; page 149). Others take a different view, whereby social defeat can be understood as an induced mind-set with a close similarity to learned helplessness. There is ethnographic evidence that defeat is part of the experience of living with a mental illness, but this might be a consequence, not a cause. It is not entirely clear that children living in inner-city poverty have more defeat experiences than anybody else, or that they experience a special form of social defeat. There is a plausible argument that entire communities are defeated and that the psychological stance of social defeat, if it is an important factor, is induced through a defeated sub-culture.

Defeated animals

The neuro-physiological consequences of defeat have been explored in animals (Björkqvist, 2001). These animal models may or may not be relevant to social defeat in humans. Defeated rats show signs of 'depression', reduced testosterone levels, reduced immune function, impaired corticosteroid responses, characteristic hormonal and neurotransmitter responses, and dominance of the sympathetic autonomic nervous system. These are not happy rats.

Defeat in rats leads to dopaminergic hyperactivity and behavioural sensitisation, with increased responses to dopamine agonists. Functional neuro-receptor imaging studies in humans show similar changes to dopaminergic pathways in people with schizophrenia who have never had antipsychotic medication. This is a somewhat tenuous evidential pathway, although a handful of studies in humans with social defeat do show some evidence for impaired endocrine function (Selten & Cantor-Graae, 2005). These circumstantial findings lend some support to the relevance of social defeat without being conclusive. They offer no evidence to suggest that it is specifically social defeat that matters.

Bullying

Psychological studies show that children who report being bullied at school are more likely to be depressed, to suffer from poor self-esteem, to feel like failures, and to experience anxiety. However, these findings are not from prospective studies. Poor self-esteem may lead to a low threshold for feeling bullied. Poor self-esteem may attract victimisation by bullies. In adults, bullying at work has been shown to lead to depression, post-traumatic stress disorder, social phobia, anxiety, loss of self-esteem, psychosomatic disturbance, and sleep problems (Björkqvist, 2001). It seems self-evident that bullying is a social defeat experience. A large proportion of the population have some experience of being bullied, and there can be little doubt that some individuals are victimised by bullies over long periods of times, with adverse consequences for their mental health. However, bullying is not necessarily associated with social deprivation. Some British public schools (where the pupils board during term-time) have harboured notorious bullying cultures, fictionally depicted from Thomas Hughes' book *Tom Brown's Schooldays* to Lindsay Anderson's film *If*. Indeed, one South American study showed that bullying was commoner in higher socio-economic groups (Chaux *et al.*, 2009).

Schizophrenia and defeat

It is argued in support of the social defeat hypothesis that it might account for some established epidemiological patterns in the incidence of schizophrenia. Schizophrenia is more common amongst the residents of larger, more competitive cities. Social competition generates social winners, and where there are winners there must be a larger number of losers. The perception of negative attitudes in others is an early or prodromal feature of psychosis, and this might provide a bridge between social defeat and paranoid thinking (Salokangas *et al.*, 2009).

People who are disadvantaged in a range of different ways are at increased risk of developing schizophrenia, including migrants, those with intellectual impairment, those with hearing problems and people with a history of childhood abuse. Understanding this in terms of social defeat might account for some of the findings amongst UK Black Minority Ethnic populations. It is suggested that there might be an increased effect of social defeat in second-generation migrants due to a much stronger element of humiliation and shame in the experience of racism and disadvantage when people reside in the country of their birth. Where there is greater social cohesion and strong social networks amongst migrant groups, one would predict less experience of social defeat. This might explain the lower prevalence of schizophrenia amongst Asians in the United Kingdom, Turks in the Netherlands, and amongst Black people living in areas where migrant groups exist as a high proportion of the local population. The higher risk amongst migrants from developing countries could reflect a higher risk of social defeat in an unfamiliar and alien urban environment. Migrants from developed countries might be protected by common socio-cultural elements between their country of origin and the host social environment. This could help them to negotiate social competition and conflict in their new community. It is not suggested that social defeat is either necessary or sufficient to cause mental illness. In any model that involves social or psychological factors, there is still a potential role for genetic and other factors.

Mental illness might involve an avalanche of defeat. Those individuals within a defeated population who become ill may experience further social defeat, more illness and a vicious spiral of deterioration. This corresponds in some respects to the concept of constellations of disadvantage in Chapter 3, where causations do not flow in one direction. Causes and consequences loop back upon each other and have multiple effects. Advocates of a more linear version of the biopsychosocial model suggest that a social factor (disadvantage) leads to a psychological consequence (social defeat) that causes a disturbance in dopamine function with sensitisation and/or increased baseline activity in the mesolimbic dopamine system, and that the result is psychosis.

Obstetric complications

Obstetric complications have long been postulated as an important contributor to the genesis of schizophrenia. It is well established that there is an effect on the risk of developing schizophrenia attributable to perinatal disadvantage (Clarke *et al.*, 2006). Poor uptake of antenatal care and obstetric complications are common in inner-city areas, and it is tempting to make a link between inner-city birth, obstetric complications and high rates of schizophrenia. However, this cannot account for the increased risk associated with inner-city birth. Twenty-five to thirty per cent of the general population have been exposed to obstetric complications, and the majority of people with schizophrenia had uncomplicated births. The pooled Odds Ratio for developing schizophrenia in people with a history of obstetric complications is about 2, which is similar to other causes of neurological disadvantage.

There are a number of different types of obstetric complication, although each type is associated with the others. Foetal growth retardation, whether expressed as low birth weight, small head circumference or small-for-gestational-age, is a consistent risk factor for schizophrenia. In same-sex twins discordant for schizophrenia, low birth weight and smaller head circumference are associated with schizophrenia, suggesting that foetal growth restriction is a risk factor independent of genetic or social factors.

Perinatal hypoxia causes structural brain abnormalities, and there is a suggestion that foetuses at high risk of developing schizophrenia may be at higher risk of sustaining hypoxic cerebral damage when exposed to perinatal adversity. In other words, a genetic vulnerability may increase the risk of perinatal brain damage and it may be the resultant cerebral damage that increases the risk of schizophrenia.

Some types of obstetric problems and complications are not routinely recorded in medical records, for example, prenatal maternal stress, prenatal infection, and intrauterine malnutrition (including vitamin deficiency), which makes it difficult to estimate how important they might be. Research is now focussing on wider obstetric disadvantage (for example, Kinney *et al.*, 2009).

There is good evidence from birth cohort studies that people who develop schizophrenia as adults tend to display a range of indicators of developmental problems during early childhood. Summarising this literature, Welham and colleagues (Welham *et al.*, 2009) concluded that the developmental trajectory of individuals who develop schizophrenia differs from the general population. From early life they show behavioural disturbances and psychopathology, intellectual and language deficits, and motor development delays. Some studies have identified alterations in language development, educational performance and physical growth.

Although the evidence on obstetric complications is inconclusive in so far as the effects appear to be largely non-specific, there have been extensive efforts to link genetic and obstetric risk (for example, Mittal *et al.*, 2008). As obstetric and perinatal risks tend to cluster, the effects of each type of risk is difficult to separate. For example, the effects of foetal hypoxia are two to three times as great in cases where the foetus is small for gestational age. The obstetric evidence may reflect another form of the constellation of disadvantage phenomenon.

Air pollution

Inner cities tend to suffer from poor air quality and heavy levels of road traffic, so it is not surprising that it has been suggested that air pollution might account for the high prevalence of psychosis in these areas. It is known that some historical road traffic contaminants, such as lead, are neuro-toxic, so that the suggestion is not completely outlandish. However, there are very few studies specifically looking for an association between schizophrenia and air pollution. Pedersen and colleagues (Pedersen *et al.*, 2004) suggested that the level of traffic pollution at the resident address at the time of birth might explain some of the urban–rural differences in schizophrenia risk. They used data from a large cohort study of children (7,455 individuals) that had the primary aim of identifying causal associations between cancer and air pollution. They took the air-pollution exposure data from this study and linked it to the Danish Psychiatric Central Register. They classified urbanisation at five levels (capital, capital suburb, provincial city, provincial town, rural area) and looked at four markers of pollution (benzene, carbon dioxide, oxides of nitrogen [NO_x] and nitrogen dioxide [NO_2]). Twenty-nine people developed schizophrenia in the follow-up period, which meant that the study had very limited statistical power. Nonetheless, they found that there was an association between schizophrenia and higher traffic densities, and benzene and carbon monoxide levels at residence of birth. These associations were stronger than the association with urbanicity per se, though the classification of urbanicity that they used was not closely linked to deprivation. There was no relationship between schizophrenia and pollution by oxides of nitrogen. Oxides of nitrogen are general air pollutants, whereas benzene and carbon monoxide are more specific emissions from motor vehicles. The findings suggest that if pollution is relevant at all, it is road traffic pollution rather than general air pollution that is the candidate toxic factor.

The problem with the hypothesis that air pollution mediates the effect of urban deprivation is precisely the association between being poor and living in less desirable environments, which includes highly polluted areas. Whilst this might provide an explanation of high levels of exposure to pollution, it is also a relationship that confounds purely epidemiological evidence. If many aspects of inner-city environments are deteriorated and undesirable, each of them will be associated with the others, and each will look like a potential causal factor when examined in isolation, owing to statistical confounding.

Toxoplasmosis

The idea that the domestic cat might be the vector for the transmission of schizophrenia in humans sounds like a satirical proposition. We find it impossible to resist linking it to the suggestion that eating fish (or more specifically fish oils) might be helpful for people diagnosed with schizophrenia (Peet & Horobin, 2002). Nonetheless, it is a serious suggestion that deserves proper consideration. As is often the case with really intriguing ideas, once you get past the apparent ridiculousness of the suggestion, it has more merit than one might suppose (Yolken et al., 2009).

Cats are the primary host of *Toxoplasma gondii* (Montoya & Liesenfeld, 2004). This is a protozoan parasite that can infect more or less all warm-blooded animals, and it causes disease in humans. In developed countries with temperate climates it is mainly transmitted by ingestion of material that has been contaminated with cat faeces. Infected meat is an important vector worldwide. It is estimated that one third of the world's population are, or have been, infected by *Toxoplasma*, but there are wide variations between countries. Seroprevalence of antibodies to *Toxoplasma gondii* in the USA is between 10 and 22.5%, but in El Salvador seroprevalence is 75%.

A number of studies have found a higher seroprevalence amongst people with schizophrenia compared to controls. A meta-analysis (Torrey et al., 2007) produced an aggregated Odds Ratio of 2.73. People with schizophrenia have a higher level of exposure to cats in childhood than controls do. There have also been studies that purport to show that men who are seropositive for *Toxoplasma* display psychological features that might correspond to a risk state for schizophrenia (or perhaps a prodromal form of the illness) (Flegr et al., 2003).

It is said that the epidemiology of schizophrenia and toxoplasmosis have similarities. These include the fact that toxoplasmosis is commoner in people with a family history of infection. As such it can be said to be pseudo-genetic. The two conditions had a similar peak age of onset, in the mid-twenties. Both have a somewhat later onset in women. In males the median age is 28 years for schizophrenia and for toxoplasmosis it is 27.7 years. The figures for women are 31.8 years and 31.9 years, respectively. Both conditions are more common in poorer and over-crowded households. There is an increased risk of stillbirths in mothers with both conditions.

There are also important differences. Toxoplasmosis is no commoner in urban than rural settings. The historical trends for the two conditions are markedly different, with a sharp fall in population seroprevalence of toxoplasmosis in the USA and Europe in the past 40 years. Schizophrenia may or may not be becoming less common, but any change in incidence is far less marked than changes in toxoplas-mosis. Countries with much higher levels of seroprevalence of toxoplasmosis do not have a greater prevalence of schizophrenia.

Toxoplasmosis is well recognised to cause a neurological disease, the symptoms of which closely resemble acute schizophrenia. In a further twist, some antipsy-chotic drugs are toxic to parasites, including *Toxoplasma gondii*. By way of experi-mental evidence, toxoplasmosis results in elevated levels of dopamine in infected laboratory animals.

Despite all of this circumstantial evidence, the case for a causal role for *Toxo-plasma Gondii* in schizophrenia is only, at best, suggestive. Although there are some persuasive advocates of the possibility, as with other causal hypotheses the evidence at this stage remains far from convincing. Even if *Toxoplasma* infection is hypothe-sised to account for just a proportion of cases of schizophrenia, there are many out-standing issues that need to be resolved before one could make a scientifically robust case. There are questions over the role of different strains of infection; whether exposure to kittens is more important than exposure to adult cats; the timing of infection; and the role of susceptibility factors. There is a substantial possibility that the entire association is due to confounding effects of social factors.

Drawing it together

We have not attempted to present a complete review of the various models that have been invoked to account for the impact of social factors on the risk that individuals develop a mental illness. All plausible models of causation of mental illness are of necessity multi-factorial. No model has sufficient explanatory power to account for all findings despite decades of intense research. There is very little unequivo-cal evidence in the form of established pathophysiological or psychopathological mechanisms. The fact that dopamine is involved in psychosis is one of the few consistent and generally accepted findings, and even this is of limited significance when taken on its own. It is pertinent to ask whether it is possible to draw anything useful from the research findings on mechanisms.

Jim Van Os is a Dutch psychiatrist who is a major contributor to the literature on schizophrenia and urbanicity. His work has some distinctive themes. For exam-ple, Van Os has conducted work on the population prevalence of psychosis-like symptoms. He seems to regard these as *forme fruste* psychotic symptoms, a partial expression of psychotic vulnerability. He appears to believe that the vulnerability is predominantly genetic, but that this is strongly influenced by social factors that are particularly prevalent in urban environments.

With Krabbendam, he has commented on what they describe as the clues to the nature of the agent or agents involved in the increased risk of schizophrenia associated with urbanicity (Krabbendam & Van Os, 2005). Firstly, they conclude that it is environmental, and that risk is based on continuous or repeated exposure (a dose effect). Secondly, they conclude that the exposure exerts its influence during childhood and adolescence, prior to the onset of the full-blown disorder. Thirdly, they conclude that it is not phenotypically silent, and that at-risk mental states are also increased. In other words, *forme fruste* psychotic symptoms are also more common amongst individuals exposed to the relevant social risk factors. Fourthly, they maintain that risk is not mediated by neuropathological impairment, traffic air pollution, childhood social position, or obstetric complications. The adverse effect of urban childhood has been increasing, and the impact is greater in cohorts born more recently. This might or might not reflect changes in the social environment in inner cities. The increase in urban risk is not compatible with postulated infective factors such as *Toxoplasma*, which is decreasing in the USA and Europe. The adverse impact of urbanicity is greater for younger rather than older persons.

Some parts of Krabbendam and Van Os's arguments are contentious, and Van Os's views on other subjects are equally strong and therefore prone to controversy. For example, he has been much more impressed by the strength of the evidence regarding schizophrenia and cannabis than we are (see Chapter 5) and he has argued for stronger controls over the availability of the drug.

Molecular genetics have brought us to a place where it seems that the likeliest model to explain the genetic evidence with regard to schizophrenia is that there is a sum total large effect from the combination of influence from many genes of small effect. It may be that the impact of inner-city poverty on the risk of schizophrenia is similar. It is hard to deny that a wide range of factors have some influence, but there is no single factor that has an effect of such strength that it comes close to accounting for the huge impact of growing up poor in a city. It is possible that some factors interact with each other in such a way that their effects multiply, rather than being additive. The sum of many small risk factors may reach tip-over point in certain types of urban environment, causing a cascade and huge increase in risk. There is, however, another possibility, which is that the reductionist biopsychosocial model has led us up a blind alley. It may be urban poverty itself that is irreducibly the factor that is toxic to the future mental health of children.

Waiting for a paradigm shift

Notwithstanding the continuous strident criticisms of psychiatry over 60 years, from the Church of Scientology and Thomas Szasz to post-psychiatry and the psycho-spirituality lobby, there is no reason to be negative about the status of psychiatry as an applied science. A huge body of scientific knowledge and evidence has accumulated regarding mental illness. A great deal is known about the interventions and the care that can help people to recover, or experience relief, from the effects of these illnesses. Our careers in mental health stretch back to the late 1970s. Since that time, many aspects of psychiatric treatment have improved markedly, though there remains a great deal to be achieved. Mental health services are far from perfect, but the awful back-wards of large mental hospitals are gone.

As a scientific community we find ourselves in a very awkward place as far as our theoretical models are concerned. There is no generally accepted theoretical stance that can comfortably explain most of what is known. We are rich in information but poor in theoretical understanding. It is not possible to make reliable predictions on the likely helpfulness of newly devised technologies and interventions. Indeed, new interventions routinely prove to be far less effective than expected, which may demonstrate a significant problem with the utility of the theories available to us.

The biopsychosocial model

Organised psychiatry likes to say that it follows a biopsychosocial model. The concept has proven popular as a defence against the complaint that psychiatry is intrinsically mechanistic, lacking in human empathy and coldly clinical, a characterisation that is often labelled the '*medical model*'. The biopsychosocial model is an attempt to emphasise psychiatry as a discipline that is scientifically ecumenical. However, the biopsychosocial model is also a meta-model of human functioning and disease. It is an attempt to accommodate to the idea that psychiatrists and other mental health professionals operate within three distinct theoretical frameworks that cannot be comfortably reconciled under a larger theoretical umbrella.

In their purest forms, current biological, psychological and social theories of mental illness are irreconcilable. Although it is not very often stated, each of them is only sustainable through ignoring conflicting evidence and rejecting ideas from the other two. Biological psychiatry tends to emphasise the primacy of molecular and genetic factors, the psychological and the social being directly determined by these (or perhaps modulating these primary effects). Some psychological theories understand biological changes as epiphenomena of psychological events. Many social theories understand mental disorders as social constructions of deviance, sometimes denying that the concept of 'mental illness' has any objective validity at all. The most strident advocates of each position sustain their arguments through a-priori denial of the validity of the other approaches, or by dismissing or rationalising away the evidence that contradicts their preferred position.

Extensive efforts have been made to link biological, psychological and social knowledge, with varying degrees of success. It would be wrong to suggest that a substantial proportion of mental health practitioners have a doctrinaire attachment to one orientation or the other. Most clinical psychiatrists in the United Kingdom and elsewhere aspire to have skills based in all three modalities. However, in practice this entails moving between three rather different ways of understanding things. It is possible to draw all three together into a coherent understanding of an individual patient's problems. However, it is much more difficult to draw all three together into a coherent theoretical understanding of the nature of mental disorder in scientific terms. Indeed, many theories are unpersuasive because they are reminiscent of efforts to scientifically prove the truth of religious texts. They involve selective use of evidence, reify the circumstantial, ignore logical errors and fail to appropriately weigh the uncertainties in the evidence against the explanatory strength of the theory. In short, true belief in a single theory is dependent on faith.

Until recently, the status of the biopsychosocial model was unassailable within Western psychiatry. It was rarely, if ever, questioned. Modern critics have tended to accuse organised psychiatry of having betrayed the holistic promise of the model, either through being too scientific (and/or in the thrall of the pharmaceutical industry)(Bracken & Thomas, 2009; Poole & Higgo, 2009) or through having lost contact with the ghost in the machine by excluding spirituality and religion from clinical practice (Poole & Cook, 2011). Now there is the beginning of a sense that the model itself may not be a model at all, and that the aspiration of holism in psychiatry might not be appropriate (Ghaemi, 2009; Cook *et al.*, 2012).

Intellectual rigour in the face of uncertainty

It seems quite clear to us that psychiatric science is presently in the position described by Thomas Kuhn as the prelude to a paradigm shift or a scientific revolution (Kuhn, 1996). It is not that scientific progress has ceased; far from it, 'normal science' trundles on, but the contradictions in the evidence cannot be reconciled, and our overall understanding has been stuck in one unsatisfactory place for some considerable time.

We should immediately state that we cannot offer novel ideas that might lead to a paradigm shift in psychiatry. It is in the nature of scientific revolutions that they can take a long time to come around. For example, Hippocrates, Galen and other classical scholars developed humoural theory, whereby the body was controlled by the balance of blood, phlegm, black bile and yellow bile within it. This theoretical dead end remained the dominant paradigm in European medicine until it was swept away in the eighteenth and nineteenth centuries by the advances that followed the adoption of the mechanistic reductionist paradigm. The inadequacies of humoural theory were already well known, having been identified by Arabic scholars (and others) centuries earlier.

In our opinion, intellectual rigour demands that the problems with psychiatry's theoretical stance should be acknowledged and the need for a paradigm shift recognised. In order to help people in the here and now, it is necessary to operate pragmatically within the uneasy biopsychosocial compromise. As clinicians and scientists who have a primary interest in the social, we are not dismissive of the importance of biological and psychological theories and advances, but we do doubt claims that they have an overarching explanatory power. Clinicians and policy makers have to use whatever approaches are helpful to patients, and even committed social psychiatrists have to use psychological and biological approaches within their preferred social orientation.

Given this unsatisfactory situation with regard to theory, practitioners have to protect their patients' best interests. In particular, they have to avoid the extrapolation of flawed theoretical frameworks to support measures that are plainly wrong at a human level. Such thinking led psychiatry to involvement in eugenic measures in the first half of the twentieth century. Darwinism had generated a very important scientific insight, but the implications of it, and the details of its mechanisms, were poorly understood. Psychiatrists participated in atrocities in Nazi Germany (Lifton, 1986), and the USA and UK also saw pseudo-scientific excesses, such as forced sterilisations, in the name of eugenics. These can only be described as crimes, and they had a basis in bad science.

This history casts a shadow over the mental health professions that cannot and should not be ignored. We are not suggesting that British psychiatry is systematically involved in seriously dubious science, but some individual practitioners continue to overestimate the scientific robustness of their ideas. On this basis they make clinical decisions that defy common sense and which are sometimes damaging to patients. Scientific rigour is not an abstract virtue. It is an essential protection for society and for individual patients. It is incumbent upon practitioners to defend their scientific and ethical integrity by reference to transparent principles that can be applied to scientific theory, empirical evidence and clinical practice.

Science versus irrationality

Notwithstanding the limitations of extant knowledge, we strongly reject a scientific nihilism that says that mental illness is too complicated to ever be properly explained. There is no need for recourse to irrationality in theoretical understanding, whether in the form of post-psychiatry (Bracken & Thomas, 2005) or through a paradigm shift to embrace the metaphysical, such as Culliford's psycho-spirituality (Culliford, 2011).

Psychiatry's claim to special expertise in helping people with mental disorders rests solely on its status as an applied science, combined with an ethical doctrine of beneficence. Science is a human endeavour, and as such it is unavoidably value-laden. One could occupy several volumes in a dissection of the core values of science, but for current purposes these could reasonably be said to include:

- The belief that the material world can be understood by human beings without reference to ineffable mysteries.
- The understanding that the available knowledge of any time can only be partial.
- The recognition that a-priori assumptions are frequently necessary, but that they should be identifiable so that they can be challenged. Recourse to an a-priori

assumption that cannot be challenged indicates that one has moved outside of the field of science.

- The following absolute criteria: theories should be testable; theories should not only explain what happens but should also predict what will happen; and that contradictory evidence must either be explained, or new theories must be developed.

This list excludes a number of features that are commonly held to be characteristic of science, such as the reduction of complex phenomena to a number of smaller and simpler processes, and the use of technology. These are tools of science, a way of making progress, rather than intrinsic components of it. For example, Occam's razor (the principle that the simplest possible explanation is likely to be correct) has proven a very useful tool across the whole arena of scientific endeavour, but there are circumstances where it can be unreliable or misleading.

The most important values that should underpin the science and the clinical practice of psychiatry are intellectual rigour and intellectual honesty. These terms themselves have a number of different meanings, but the fundamental idea is that one should aspire to maintain consistency, scepticism and independent mindedness; that one's attachment to a set of ideas should be proportional to the evidence supporting them; that alternative plausible explanations should not be arbitrarily dismissed; and that the unavoidable human tendency to an emotional attachment to one's own ideas should be tempered by a more dispassionate appreciation of other possibilities. For social scientists, such as ourselves, intellectual rigour demands that we should pay serious attention to the evidence regarding the importance of biological factors in determining the course, and perhaps in causing, mental illness. This is precisely because we are least interested in the biological and are therefore most likely to make an error by ignoring it.

Pathogenic social environments

Whether or not a paradigm shift will eventually assist in understanding the totality of the evidence, there is one idea that is unusual in medical thinking that bears consideration. As mentioned in Chapter 1, it is possible that a particular type of social environment might have an emergent property that causes schizophrenia in those who grow up within it. By analogy with pathogens, such as micro-organisms, that cause specific physical diseases, such a social environment might be considered pathogenic.

This would mean that growing up in a deprived inner city exposes children to something different to disadvantaged children growing up elsewhere. It does not simply expose them to an unusually high level of individual risk factors that are evident in other environments. Most of the population, according to this idea, are exposed to a range of risk factors for schizophrenia. However, there is a qualitative difference to the additional risk factor in the inner city, which cannot be reduced to this element or that, but which is an intrinsic characteristic of these areas.

The concept of a pathogenic environment is uncomfortable, because the science we are used to depends heavily on teasing out individual factors and reducing phenomena to their component parts. It is hard to know how one might test such an idea epidemiologically or experimentally. Nonetheless, as a speculation it does have some strengths. It might explain the very high prevalence of psychosis in inner cities compared with much lower (though still elevated) levels in nearby areas that are only slightly less deprived. It might also explain some of the micro-geography of mental illness that is evident to community psychiatrists, whereby some streets or small estates have especially high levels of mental illness, independent of the effect of aggregations of social housing.

During the Industrial Revolution, there was a belief that the growth of cities was causing an epidemic of mental illness. It has frequently been noted that, given the modern prevalence of schizophrenia, there are surprisingly few descriptions of it prior to the mid eighteenth century, compared with other mental illnesses. It has sometimes been suggested that contemporaneous observations were right, that prior to the Industrial Revolution schizophrenia was rare, but that it became common in the new and rapidly growing cities of the time. In the past decade, some countries in the developing world, such as India and China, have been experiencing urbanisation at a pace that has been even more rapid than Europe experienced 200 years ago. If the idea that inner cities are a specific pathogenic environment is correct, then one would expect to see an epidemic of schizophrenia in Indian and Chinese cities over the next 20 to 30 years. There are significant barriers to the use of growth in developing countries as a kind of natural experiment. The emergent nations lack infrastructure and services, and it is difficult to accurately determine changes in the incidence of mental illness. Nonetheless, it is surely a scientific necessity to attempt to observe what happens to the mental health of people living in the emerging mega cities.

Increasing equality as a public health measure

Poverty, and attendant inequality, is associated with high levels of psychiatric morbidity. Is the position analogous to smoking and lung cancer in the 1950s? It was recognised that there was a substantial increase in risk associated with smoking long before the mechanisms were identified, and before smoking could be separated from other risk factors such as occupational exposure to some types of dust. Doctors lobbied against smoking, and some lives were saved. The argument at the time was 'How much evidence do you want?' More recently, this rationale has successfully been deployed by researchers into cannabis and schizophrenia in advising the government against decriminalisation of cannabis possession on the basis of estimated Odds Ratios of 1.4 to 1.6. These are considerably lower than the Odds Ratios associated with inner-city childhood and schizophrenia.

It is not scientifically certain that intervention to reduce poverty would have any impact on the incidence of schizophrenia. International comparisons do show national variations in the prevalence of these disorders, but they are not as great as they are for other diseases associated with poverty. It can be argued that there is adequate justification to reduce urban poverty in order to prevent psychosis, as there is no possibility of obtaining experimental evidence before taking action. Some of the most successful public health measures have been introduced on a similar basis. Adequate sanitation transformed the incidence of infectious disease in the UK long before there was any certainty that it would be successful.

Main points in this chapter

1. A range of mechanisms have been explored that might explain the relationship between inner-city childhood and adult psychosis.
2. Childhood adversity, including physical, sexual and emotional abuse, has a known association with adult psychosis.
3. Obstetric complications are a known risk factor for schizophrenia and are common amongst inner-city populations. However, the association cannot explain the size of the increased risk of psychosis in urban areas.
4. Other factors such as road traffic pollution and toxoplasmosis have been explored, but probably make only a minor contribution. The apparent relationships may be due to confounding associations with deprivation.
5. The biopsychosocial model is scientifically unsatisfactory. It will require a paradigm shift before all the evidence on causation of psychosis can be drawn together into a single convincing model.
6. There is a possibility that inner-city poverty has an emergent characteristic as a specific pathogenic environment that causes schizophrenia. This is not truly a refutable hypothesis, and it is hard to know how the possibility can be investigated.
7. It is arguable that there is sufficient evidence to justify lobbying for action to reduce inner-city deprivation on the basis that this would be likely to reduce the incidence and prevalence of psychosis.

8

Stigma

Stigma has emerged as one of the great themes in social sciences' examination of mental health. Although the concept of social stigma is not new, interest in it has exploded since the millennium. According to Bos and colleagues (Bos *et al.*, 2013), three quarters of the entire stigma literature on 'PsycInfo' has been published in the last ten years. It has become axiomatic that social stigma is one of the great issues for everyone working in the mental health field.

The concept of stigma is a metaphor based on the ancient Greek practice of branding or marking criminals, with the consequence that they were socially shunned. Similar practices persist in some parts of the world today. Stigma as a social phenomenon has no agreed definition, and on close examination it is complicated. In particular, the relationship between disadvantage and stigma is far from straightforward.

Is stigma the most useful construct?

Understanding and challenging the stigma associated with mental illness has become a core element of the work of mental health organisations, including the charity MIND and the Royal College of Psychiatrists. Stigma and stigmatising attitudes are identified by services users to be amongst the most difficult aspects of having a mental illness. We have large-scale public education campaigns that have ambitious objectives of reducing discrimination against people with mental disorders. For example, Time to Change is a campaign with public and voluntary sector funding, led by two mental health charities in the UK. It commenced in 2007 and it is due to continue until 2015. It has specific targets of reducing measurable discrimination against people with mental health problems and increasing their social capital. It is entirely laudable that organisations put their money where their mouth is in this way, in order to try to tackle a real problem that troubles many people diagnosed with mental illness.

However, the effects of stigma vary for people with different diagnoses, from different backgrounds and living in different social environments. For example, Stephen Fry is a British writer, television presenter and actor. He has quite bravely disclosed his mental health problems to the public, together with the explanation that these may be due to bipolar affective disorder. This had the positive effect of opening up public debate and discussion about mental illness. As a consequence, he is the current president of MIND. The disclosure has had no discernible adverse effect on Fry's reputation; it may even have enhanced his public standing. The same is not true for Frank Bruno, a Black British celebrity and former boxer. Details of Bruno's mental health problems, apparently related to bipolar affective disorder, were forcibly and sensationally exposed in the tabloid press in 2003 when he was reported to have been detained under the Mental Health Act. In a headline the *Sun* newspaper described him as 'Bonkers Bruno'. Although there was public outrage over tasteless and inappropriate reporting, the episode served to reinforce negative stereotypes of both mental illness and Black people.

Bruno is a supporter of the Time to Change campaign. He has retained his status as a public figure, but the two disclosures arose in different contexts and their stigmatising impact was very different. Both stories might have had another quality if the disorder concerned had been schizophrenia rather than bipolar affective disorder. However, it is difficult to avoid the conclusion that stigma in these cases was not embedded in the concept of 'bipolar affective disorder'. It seems to have been more closely related to reported behaviours and other characteristics of the person than the mental illness per se. This is congruent with the research evidence, which suggests that whilst a mental illness label has an impact on stigma, other characteristics, including perceived dangerousness, are also important (Martin *et al.*, 2000).

There are a number of problems with the concept of stigma, especially if the main purpose in identifying and understanding it is to overcome the effects of disadvantage and discrimination. There are other ways of thinking about inequality that may prove more useful. Struggles to overcome discrimination tend to be successful where they are led from within marginalised groups. Examples include the civil rights and anti-racist movements, the women's movement and the gay rights movement. There are few examples of successful paternalistic campaigns against discrimination, as these tend to reinforce the idea that marginalised groups are helpless and ineffectual. This does little to challenge their stigmatised status.

The modern service user movement has a strong voice that has made some real progress in changing public perceptions (Beresford, 2010). It has much in common with other activist movements, and it is arguable that it is effective because it challenges power relationships. No matter how well intended anti-stigma campaigns by the Royal College of Psychiatrists might be (Crisp *et al.*, 2005), the power differential between psychiatrists and their patients, together with psychiatrists' primary focus on symptoms of mental illness and on risk, is always likely to undermine their effectiveness.

Stigma is difficult to define and isolate. It is hard to separate the stigma of mental illness from the stigma of those social characteristics associated with mental illness, such as low socio-economic status, substance misuse and long-term unemployment. The social context of the person is important in understanding the effects of stigma. These do not arise in isolation. Stigma is dynamic and multifaceted. Poverty itself is stigmatised and it is frequently construed by policy makers to be a consequence of bad choices or indolence. Similarly, alcohol-related harm is construed as a consequence of irresponsible drinking, a bad choice, rather than an inevitable consequence of the availability of very cheap alcohol. Young Black men are stereotyped as criminal and aggressive. Poverty, substance misuse and minority ethnicity are all associated with major mental illness. The stereotypes associated with these characteristics cannot be isolated from the stigma of a label of mental illness.

There is a peculiar phenomenon whereby victimhood is increasingly adopted as an explanatory framework for the vagaries of everyday life. The fact that there are groups of people who unequivocally have been victimised does not imply that victimisation is the most useful way to understand the full range of adverse human experience. Post-traumatic stress disorder (PTSD) was originally understood to arise where people survived exceptional and life-threatening danger. It was first clearly identified in American veterans from the Vietnam War (Summerfield, 1999). The PTSD construct has subsequently been applied to a very wide range of reactions to less extreme experiences, including chronic childhood adversity and even humiliations (Seides, 2010). There is an uncomfortable tendency to believe that victimhood validates unhappiness. For example, there is a body of work on the stigma associated with being intellectually gifted (e.g. Coleman & Cross, 2005). Whilst it is clear that individual high ability can carry significant disadvantages, it is problematic to regard the disadvantages of being very clever as the same as, or similar to, the disadvantages of having a chronic mental illness. In both cases, understanding these experiences solely in terms of externally imposed stigma may not adequately acknowledge the complexity of disadvantage, and the potential strategies to challenge and overcome it.

Is stigma an epiphenomenon of de-institutionalisation?

Erving Goffman was a highly influential social scientist, best known in psychiatry for his work on 'total institutions' (Goffman, 1961). He was also an early and important contributor to the development of the modern concept of social stigma (Goffman, 1963). Goffman stated that stigma arose when individuals bore characteristics that damaged their identity permanently and prevented their full participation in society. To Goffman, stigma was an attribute that spoiled an individual's identity. He identified three main types: defects of the body, such as cerebral palsy; defects of character, including mental illness; and membership of socially devalued groups such as extreme political or religious groups, or ethnic minorities. Goffman's ideas about stigma have influenced and shaped much modern thinking on the subject.

Although Goffman was a sociologist, the concept of stigma truly belongs to social psychology. Disadvantage is understood in terms of psychological and cultural processes that have the effect of consigning some people with recognisable characteristics (in this case a mental illness diagnosis or behaviours that suggest such a diagnosis) to a shunned 'out' group. From the late 1950s, Goffman, R.D. Laing (Laing, 1965) and others started to re-evaluate the position of people who were suffering from long-term severe mental illnesses and who in those days tended to reside in large mental hospitals. It is relevant that this re-evaluation occurred against the background of the beginnings of de-institutionalisation. Large numbers of people were being discharged from institutions. In part, this was due to the introduction and widespread deployment of new antipsychotic drugs such as chlorpromazine. More importantly, there was a new realisation that it was possible to care for people with mental illness outside of a hospital setting and that this was often cheaper and more satisfactory than inpatient care (Mandelbrote & Folkard, 1961).

It is orthodox social science teaching to say that Goffman and Laing provided a radical critique that challenged many of the fundamentals of psychiatry. Goffman dissected the inhumane and brutalising conditions under which people with chronic mental illness were nursed in large mental hospitals. Laing challenged the idea that the things that people with schizophrenia say are meaningless and that the condition is psychologically unintelligible. Fifty years later, both are acknowledged by mainstream psychiatry, and it is possible to see that whilst their writings did have a significant impact, neither of them was as far from the mainstream as it might have appeared.

Firstly, whilst both were pursuing an agenda to liberate people under psychiatric treatment, they had little option but to regard their subjects as oppressed and broken. Their position was paternalistic and, in Laing's case, remained so in his efforts to establish a new type of mental institution at Kingsley Hall (Crossley, 1998). They studied patients as passive subjects in much the same way as conventional mental health researchers of the time. This was a liberation where the liberated had no active role. The de-institutionalisation that accompanied their work was not a response to a clamour amongst patients. In fact, some hospital residents did not wish to leave hospital, though relatively few missed institutional life once they had been resettled (Trauer et al., 2001).

Secondly, de-institutionalisation commenced in the UK from about 1952, long before the new drug treatments became generally available (Rogers & Pilgrim, 2001). Many factors contributed to this. The mental hospitals had been taken from local authority control in 1948 and became part of the newly formed NHS. The Second World War had brought new therapeutic optimism and enthusiasm for biological and social interventions. Demobilisation of military doctors had given mental health services a larger, younger medical workforce. The years after the war brought waves of disclosure about the horrors of concentration camps and death camps under Nazi and Soviet regimes. Dehumanising institutions were regarded with a new suspicion.

Consequently, the belief that mental hospital care was the best option for people with chronic mental illness was under challenge from within the institutions themselves. Progressive medical superintendents led rapid reforms in mental hospitals (Clark, 1996). De-institutionalisation was a radical idea compared with the pre-War consensus, but it was not necessarily radical in the sense of conflicting with the new ideas that had been embraced by the psychiatric mainstream. Both Laing and Goffman can be understood to have been pushing against open doors. The objective of closing mental hospitals and resettling people in the community was enthusiastically embraced by Enoch Powell when he was Minister of Health in a Conservative government between 1960 and 1963.

Stigma and mental illness became part of the scientific literature as people with unresolved severe mental health problems were resettled in communities that were ill-prepared and unwelcoming. Suburban communities found group homes and hostels opening in their neighbourhoods. During the preceding 150 years, people displaying conspicuously odd behaviour had been removed from public view through the asylum system. The general population had no framework for understanding people who seemed unpredictable in their behaviour. Local populations became concerned about the possibility that these newcomers might show inappropriate aggressive or sexual behaviour, and that they might have an unnatural interest in children. Whilst such reactions were not universal, they were not rare. Freedom from the restrictions of life in the mental hospital could be accompanied by recurrent taunting and exclusion from shops and pubs. Stigma and resistance to resettlement was a problem for those responsible for the management of mental health care and it remains so today (Link *et al.*, 1999). This has had some impact in focusing the anti-stigma agenda on public education. This is an arena that is familiar and comfortable for public authorities and it is less troubling than attempting to directly address issues of employment and integration.

What causes stigma?

We can settle upon a functional concept of stigma that goes beyond mere stereotyping. The importance of stigma is the extent to which it makes the lives of people with mental illness difficult. Early debates about stigma focussed on the question of whether the diagnostic label was the vector of stigma (in keeping with the ideas of Thomas Szasz and others who believed that psychiatric diagnoses simply marginalised and decontextualised deviant behaviour) or whether stigma was due to the abnormal or unusual behaviour of people with mental illness. The conclusion of this debate appears to be that both have some impact.

There is an optimistic theory that suggests that stigma can reasonably easily be tackled through education, because stigma arises from ignorance. According to this theory, the general population has little understanding of mental illness, and they are therefore prey to atavistic fears about madness. Once properly educated, people will come to see that the realities of mental illness are different to their fears, and stigma will fall away. This type of theory has driven the programmes of public education mentioned above. Unfortunately, the current evidence does not support this view.

There has been a general consensus that stigma has been slowly decreasing since de-institutionalisation started in the 1950s. Some right-wing commentators (e.g. Scruton, 2000) have lamented the reduction of stigma in general as a reflection of the loss of the moral dimension in national life. It is only recently that there have been efforts to assess empirically whether stigma really is lessening. In the USA there is a long-standing government programme to survey population attitudes, the General Social Survey. From 1996, questions were included on attitudes to mental illness. Pescosolido has published extensively on public attitudes to mental illness (Pescosolido, 2013). She has used General Social Survey data to assess alterations in public attitudes between 1996 and 2006, together with data from other sources. She found that there has been a significant improvement in the general population's understanding of mental illness over a long period of time. Most of the population are familiar with the main diagnoses of psychiatry. They recognise the difference between mental illness and problems of everyday life. There is a good awareness of the treatments that are available for mental disorders. However, according to Pescosolido the diagnoses still carry negative connotations and stigma. Over the years, the dominant explanations held by the general public have progressively shifted away from the psychosocial towards the biological, in keeping with the same trend in American psychiatry. The evidence suggests that the belief that mental illnesses have a neurobiological basis is particularly associated with negative ideas and with the idea that mental illness is permanent (Pescosolido et al., 2010). In other words, greater knowledge does not necessarily dissipate stigma.

Pescosolido also reports that attitudes linking mental illness to acts of violence have not decreased, and may have increased. High-school shootings have had some negative impact on attitudes to children with mental health problems (Pescosolido et al., 2007). When asked open-ended questions, people frequently spontaneously cite wordings from policy documents and mental health legislation which frame the grounds for compulsory treatment. They use terms such as 'dangerous to self and others'. These are understood to encapsulate some essential quality of mental illness. In other words, wordings that were intended to limit the scope of compulsory treatment have come to be seen by a section of the general public to capture a core feature of mental illness.

One way of understanding stigma is that it is a consequence of the need of social groups to define themselves and set their boundaries. This view says that all stable social structures, whether families, organisations or neighbourhood communities, must have a means of identifying those who are *other*. Without this, membership of the social group is indistinct and group integrity is threatened. The in-group is marked by similarity, or at least by the perception of similarity.

One of Sir Winston Churchill's great achievements was to articulate a sense of solidarity and determination amongst the British people during the Second World War, best captured by his use of the phrase 'our island race'. This was underpinned by the existence of an extremely threatening foe or out-group in the form of the Nazi regime in Germany. However, the perception that the British Isles were occupied by a homogenous 'island race' would have been a little ridiculous if the circumstances had not been so desperate. Long before mass Commonwealth immigration, the United Kingdom was characterised by cultural, linguistic and ethnic diversity. A Cockney cab driver and a Shetland smallholder would struggle to understand each other's speech, let alone identify much in common in their lifestyle or circumstances. The perception of belonging to a single group, an island race, arose largely from an awareness of who was excluded from it, namely the Germans and their allies.

Under everyday circumstances, signs of disturbing difference, of *otherness*, signify membership of the out-group. According to this model, there is a stereotype which indicates that mental illness leads to unpredictable and disruptive behaviour, and this is undesirable for the social group. The stigma of mental illness arises wherever there is a diagnostic label or where minor peculiarities of behaviour indicate that the person has a mental illness. These create assumptions about likely behaviour and the person is excluded from the social group. An alternative version of this model gives less emphasis to anticipated behaviour and more emphasis to atavistic fears of insanity, whereby irrationality is feared to be contagious.

Understanding social stigma and exclusion of out-groups as basic social functions of stable social groupings tends to lead to the conclusion that it is inevitable. This view broadly corresponds to the ideas of the saloon-bar bigot who justifies his prejudices on the basis that 'it's only human nature to dislike people who are different'. Buehler has captured some of the sentiment in the statement that it would take a paradigm shift to overcome the stigma of mental illness.[1] This brings us full circle whereby understanding disadvantage in terms of stigma seems to lead us to believe that disadvantage cannot be overcome.

At the other end of the explanatory spectrum, there have been attempts to understand stigma in terms of neurobiological correlates. These are largely based on functional neuro-imaging studies of people who are victims of stigma and those whose attitudes are stigmatising. Both experiences appear to be associated with activation of specific brain regions (Derks *et al.*, 2008; Amodio, 2010). Although it is possible to generate sociobiological hypotheses from such findings, taken on their own they offer no real evidence about the causes or impact of stigma. Neurobiology is important, but it is a logical fallacy to believe that brain activation is necessarily prior to, or causal of, events in the mind. Unless one adheres to mind–body dualism, brain events and mind events are the same thing and do not stand

---

[1] Buehler A (2004) Initial perceptions of labels to initial perceptions of common humanity: a paradigm shift in the disability field. www.humiliationstudies.org/documents/BuehlerLabels.pdf *retrieved 5 March 2013.*

in causal relationship to each other. Similarly, the existence of neurobiological correlates to social phenomena does not indicate that they are 'hard wired' or biological in origin.

There is sound evidence that public reporting of mental illness is dominated by news stories linking mental illness to violence, especially sudden unprovoked violence against strangers. As noted above, dangerousness has become more prominent in perceptions of mental illness amongst the general public. This has had a significant impact on policy makers across the world, who have become increasingly concerned with safety and risk. There is experimental evidence that constant reiteration of the association between mental illness and violence has been an important factor in maintaining stigma and negative attitudes to people with mental disorders in general (Philo *et al.*, 1994).

There is a real association between schizophrenia and violence at all levels of severity (Walsh *et al.*, 2002). It is hard to precisely quantify the relative risk of violence amongst people with this diagnosis, as the risk is partially attributable to confounding factors such as socio-economic status and male gender. The risk of violence amongst people with schizophrenia is modified by factors such as substance misuse that are also powerful risk factors amongst the rest of the population. The only risk factor for violence that is specific to schizophrenia is the presence of active psychotic symptoms. Whilst it cannot be denied that the increased relative risk is real, the absolute risk of violence by people with schizophrenia is low. The vast majority of people with schizophrenia and other mental illnesses are not aggressive and pose no risk to other people.

Unfortunately, the public linking of violence and mental disorder also runs in the opposite direction. In the face of acts of extreme violence, such as the massacre of Norwegian teenagers by Anders Breivik, there is a response that looks for an explanation in mental disorder. Breivik's trial was dominated by conflicting psychiatric opinions (Melle, 2013). An initial diagnosis of schizophrenia gave way to later assertions of personality disorder or neuro-developmental problems such as Asperger's or Tourette's syndromes. The debate was based on the assumption amongst professionals, courts and the public that an atrocity of this nature could not be perpetrated by someone who was 'mentally normal'. At his trial, personality disorder emerged as the most likely diagnosis. If Breivik's key personality abnormality was his capacity to commit a cold-blooded massacre for political reasons, then the personality abnormality cannot also be an explanation for his behaviour. Personality disorder and behaviour are bound together here by definition, not by causality. This is a tautology, a logical error that is profoundly embedded in social attitudes to violence. The irony is that the great genocides of the twentieth century were committed by bureaucrats and functionaries who showed little or no evidence of mental disorder of any type.

Violence and mental disorder are further linked in so far as they are both seen to be manifestations of irrationality. In fact both frequently occur in the absence of irrationality. If violence is believed to be intrinsically irrational, and if a secular society sees mental disorder as the main source of irrationality, the link is likely to be difficult to break. Psychiatry has tended to dominate scientific understanding of irrationality, although strictly speaking it is a subject more suited to the methods of experimental psychology.

The spread of risk aversion probably contributes to growing concern over violence and mental illness. It is commonplace to condemn modern attitudes to risk, with a head-shaking disapproval of children being driven to school and with the popular cri-de-coeur: 'It's health and safety gone mad!' The trouble is that the health and safety culture in the UK has saved lives. In 1981 there were 441 deaths amongst employees from industrial accidents. In 2011 there were 118 deaths.[2] This is part of a long-term downward trend. Whilst the disappearance of dangerous jobs such as mining has affected this, a more risk-averse national culture has helped avoid unnecessary fatalities. Although it is frequently said that mental health services should deploy 'creative risk taking', there is little evidence that this occurs or that those who review serious untoward incidents are sympathetic to creative risk taking when it goes wrong. In a society that dislikes risk, it is hard to see how mental health services can be excluded from risk reduction even if absolute risks are small.

Hierarchies of stigma

It has been recognised since the 1950s that some conditions carry greater stigma than others. It appears that the rank order of stigma has altered little over the past 60 years (Pescosolido, 2013). Problems of life have consistently been the least stigmatising mental health problem. Drug addiction has been the most stigmatising, with alcohol misuse a close second. Major mental illness is between these extremes. Similar hierarchies exist for disorders affecting children. The general population continues to report a greater wish to maintain a social distance from people with the most stigmatised disorders compared with people with the least stigmatised problems. They are particularly against these people marrying into their family or moving in next door.

There are hierarchies of stigma amongst people with mental disorders, and amongst professionals who work in mental health. So-called dual diagnosis is particularly problematic. This term is used to describe people who have a major mental illness and a substance misuse problem. Both of the stigmatised groups that they belong to tend to identify the problem they don't share as being the person's defining disorder. They reject communality with them as a consequence. People with dual diagnosis are regarded by both groups as belonging to the other *out-group*. Similarly, mental health professionals, organised to specialist functions, are increasingly inflexible in their ability to cope with combined or complex problems (Krayer *et al.*, 2013). Substance misuse services usually require that a mental illness

---

[2] Health and Safety Executive (2013) RIDDOR – Reporting of injuries, diseases and dangerous outcomes regulations. www.hse.gov.uk/statistics/tables/index.htm *retrieved 5 March 2013.*

is under control before they offer treatment, and mental health services can demand that substance misuse is under control before they act. There is a complex web of rejection and stigma. The person belongs to two groups that are stigmatised by the general population, and they are rejected by peers and services alike.

Protective factors

The discussion regarding Stephen Fry's public self-disclosure of mental health problems illustrates that some people can avoid personal stigma from a stigmatising diagnosis. Fry is not alone. The Time To Change website[3] lists a significant number of celebrities who support the campaign, some of whom disclose mental health problems that they, or close relatives, have suffered. Some individuals have a public persona that includes mental illness as an intrinsic element. For example, the late Syd Barrett was the original guitarist and songwriter in Pink Floyd. He also recorded two influential solo albums. His status as one of the originators of psychedelic rock music is closely linked to severe mental health problems and a reclusive lifestyle for the last 30 years of his life. The supposed link between his creative ability and his mental illness was set out in one of Pink Floyd's most celebrated songs, *Shine On You Crazy Diamond*, recorded years after he had left the band. Similarly, Spike Milligan's offbeat and surreal humour was seen to be inextricably linked to a mental illness that occasionally led him to act in unusual ways in public.

Each of these celebrities appears to have avoided stigma but none of them publicly displayed mental illness prior to their celebrity. All were of high social status when mental illness was disclosed to the public and their behaviour did not conform to common stereotypes of mental ill health. Stigma is especially likely to stick where people are already of low social status, although this does not appear to be true for all forms of stigma. It does appear to be common social currency that mental illness is not due to a personal failing or moral inadequacy. The same is not true of substance misuse, which is widely seen as being blameworthy. This may be due to the belief that people can only overcome substance misuse problems through making choices that are dependent on personal motivation. The footballer George Best, the actor Oliver Reed and the singer Amy Winehouse attracted pity and opprobrium in equal measure after public displays of drunkenness followed by premature death.

There has been some work on factors that protect individuals from the negative effects of social stigma. Corrigan and Watson (2002) have drawn on work in stigmatised groups other than people with mental illness. They suggest that most people with mental illness are aware of stigma, but there are differences in how people react to it. They speculate that there are three main reactions. One reaction is that self-esteem is diminished, with a Goffman-type damage to identity which is constantly reinforced by stigmatising attitudes in others. This group are affected by shame, and internalise the validity of stigma. For this group of people, stigma limits their life opportunities. A second group simply ignore stigma and are indifferent to it. They don't regard it as relevant to them personally and it does not materially affect their behaviour or their well-being. A third group rail against stigma and are energised by their marginalised status. This is the activist group who refuse to passively accept their position. Conceptualising stigma as an impersonal flaw in the social system seems to be relatively protective against its effects. If findings from other forms of social stigma are confirmed to be applicable to mental illness, it is important to recognise that people are not passive victims and can modify their own and other people's attitudes.

There has been some work on self-stigma, which in the literature is the tendency to internalise and accept stigma (Rusch *et al.*, 2010). It is closely linked to identity, to self-esteem and to feelings of shame and humiliation. Self-stigma shapes people's behaviour. Difficulties in inter-personal behaviour may be exacerbated by lack of self-confidence and an expectation of rejection. A low expectation of recovery can be a self-fulfilling prophecy. Stigma is a social phenomenon as well as an individual one. It affects the parents of people with mental illness (Hasson-Ohayon *et al.*, 2011), so that some people are caught in a nexus of external stigma and self-stigma.

There is evidence that identification with a stigmatised group can protect people from some of the adverse effects of stigma. Mental health support groups appear to increase participants' resistance to stigma, possibly by preventing internalisation of stereotypes by providing a supportive social milieu that rejects them. However, this is not unambiguous, and some aspects of self-esteem may be damaged by strong identification with a mental illness support group (Crabtree *et al.*, 2010).

There is another way of understanding self-stigma. People do not develop mental health problems from a neutral position. Prior to developing a mental illness, people are likely to share the same attitudes as the rest of the population. Sometimes these attitudes are highly stigmatising. The person finds themself in a bad place, suffering from a disorder that they regard as shameful and unacceptable. Negotiating a shift in personal attitudes under these circumstances can be difficult, and people in this situation can react to a mental illness diagnosis with a disproportionate nihilism that is hard to shift.

The stigma of poverty and class

There is a very substantial literature on the social stigma associated with poverty, low socio-economic status, homelessness, illiteracy and a range of problems strongly associated with poverty. Historically, a distinction was made between the deserving and the undeserving poor. Schneider and Remillard (2013) state that in previous times there was a further distinction between the honest poor, who were deserving and stoically suffered their poverty in submission to God's will, and the dishonest poor, whose poverty was divine punishment for deviance. They state that the modern discourse focusses on worthiness to receive help. Bad luck and temporary setbacks fall into the former category. Moral failings and bad lifestyle choices fall into the latter. They summarise research that shows that social contact with excluded people such as those who are homeless alters attitudes. These people move from blame to *there but for the grace of God go I*, in other words a better understanding of the ways in which impersonal pressures and structural social problems affect individuals. However, Schneider and Remillard go on to suggest that this ostensibly more liberal attitude is no less stigmatising, as it maintains the *otherness* of homeless people and encourages pity rather than a sense of common humanity. The social hierarchy between the well-meaning and the homeless is unchanged. As is common amongst commentators influenced by post-structuralists such as Foucault, they conclude that there may not be much that can be done to reduce stigma. In particular, they regard anti-stigma campaigns based upon increased knowledge as intrinsically ineffective or counter-productive.

There is an implicit belief in much of the literature that the demise of working-class institutions and social solidarity has increased the stigma of poverty. It is certainly very tempting to believe that trade unions and communities that struggled collectively to improve their lot were relatively immune from social stigma. However, there are simply no data to support this assumption, which may be wrong. The 1930s were a period of great struggle, but the workhouses were still open. We can be more certain about the impact of contemporary policy. There has been a growth in the belief that those on benefits choose not to work and that the honest tax payer is burdened by those who decide that life is more pleasant in economic inactivity whilst drawing welfare benefits (Park *et al.*, 2005). It seems as if changing stigma may require a shift in the general understanding of the relationship between structural economic problems, such as the banking crisis of 2008, and individual economic disadvantage.

Is there a way forward?

Stigma is important because it affects people's lives. It is more than one thing, and it isn't clear that it is unequivocally a bad thing. Room (2005) has pointed out that the stigma associated with criminal behaviour is appropriate. Social disapproval and a degree of individual blame in the face of criminality is inevitable if crime is to be discouraged. However, social attitudes are not so malleable as to allow stigma to attach solely to behaviours where a particular set of liberal values determine that it is appropriate. Even if this were possible, the stigma of crime would leak into attitudes to substance misuse, which has a strong association with some forms of crime.

Health education about mental illness is a worthwhile exercise in itself. It is not necessary to demonstrate reductions in stigma in order to justify such campaigns. However, it seems unlikely that it will be possible to really influence the stigma of mental illness as an isolated phenomenon. People who are stigmatised are not passive victims, and it does appear that activism by the stigmatised has greater benefits, even if these are not unambiguous.

In 2011, an English Mental Health Strategy *No Health without Mental Health* made a commitment to 'parity of esteem between mental and physical health services'. Amongst its objectives were to improve the physical health of people with a mental disorder and to promote understanding of the interaction between physical and mental health. The 'parity of esteem' terminology is awkward and peculiar, but tangible steps to integrate health care may have more impact than 'hearts and minds' campaigns. The US state of Oregon introduced 'parity' legislation to prevent insurers differentially limiting coverage for mental health and substance abuse services compared with physical health services. This was shown to have no impact on overall health costs (McConnell *et al.*, 2012). The measure tackled a consequence of stigma rather than stigma itself, which may be a more fruitful way forward. Combating tangible disadvantage is easier than attempting to dislodge complex and deeply rooted negative stereotypes. Prejudice is only potent where there is a power differential between two groups. Where there is a power differential, the absence of prejudice doesn't necessarily solve the problems of the disadvantaged. The evidence strongly suggests that if steps were taken to overcome large-scale social inequalities, the problems associated with stigma would lessen.

Main points in this chapter

1. Stigma is a metaphor for a number of different psychological and social phenomena.
2. Stigma arises in a social context. The stigma associated with mental illness is influenced by other aspects of the person including their behaviour, social class and ethnicity.
3. Theoretical models of stigma tend to lead to the conclusion that it is difficult or impossible to modify without major social change.
4. People suffering from two types of stigmatised problem, for example, people with 'dual diagnosis', may find it very difficult to secure services owing to cross-stigmatisation.
5. Efforts to challenge stigma are best led by the stigmatised. Paternalistic campaigns against stigma are intrinsically contradictory.
6. It may be more fruitful to tackle the tangible effects of stigma rather than directly trying to alter deep-seated negative stereotypes.

9

Recovery

'*Recovery*'[1] has become the dominant conceptual framework for mental health services in the twenty-first century. Recovery focuses on the lives of individual service users. It is more concerned with functionality than disability. It has deep roots in the service user movement. For this and for many other reasons it can be difficult to suggest that there might be problems with the concept of Recovery. Only the most dyed-in-the-wool reactionary would wish to align themselves with the things that Recovery seeks to overcome: hopelessness, paternalism and disadvantage. Nonetheless, whilst Recovery remains a banner under which the service user movement marches, it is also the label attached to the state-sanctioned model for mental health services in several countries, including the UK. In the absence of a universally accepted definition of Recovery, it is right to look critically at this rather loose model that has been readily adopted by governments that have an unwavering faith in free markets and who show limited commitment in other policy areas to equality and social justice.

Irrespective of the affirmative sentiments that underlie the Recovery model, it is particularly relevant to examine its application to the care of people who have serious mental illnesses that do not respond well to treatment. Many people in this situation reside in long-stay inpatient units, often behind locked doors and under the care of private companies at public expense. It is surprising to find that no one knows how many people are cared for in this way. They are part of a dispersed system of care that has been labelled 'the virtual asylum' (Poole *et al.*, 2002). In England in 2009/2010, the cost of this type of care was around £690 million (US$1067 million; €770 million) (Ryan *et al.*, 2011). Whilst it is right to emphasise that most people diagnosed with severe mental illness can and will recover, it is also important to pay due attention to the needs of people for whom Recovery is a very slow and difficult journey. It should not be denied that a small but important minority don't recover at all.

---

[1] Where 'Recovery' is capitalised we refer to the ideas of the Recovery movement. Otherwise 'recovery' has its usual meaning.

The origins of Recovery as applied to mental illness

Both the de-institutionalisation and the anti-psychiatry movements were led by psychiatrists, who published books and papers about what they were doing. The Recovery movement was initially developed and led by service users. As a consequence, its early origins were not documented and cannot be traced in academic publications in the same way. In any case, Recovery has complex and multiple origins. Whilst the most important impetus came from the service user movement, some of its origins lay within mainstream psychiatry (especially rehabilitation services), some came from anti-psychiatry, and some threads originated in self-help movements like Alcoholics Anonymous. This is not the place for a comprehensive history of the Recovery movement, but it is possible to identify some of the main conceptual threads.

There is a general consensus that, as far as the mental health professions are concerned, the Recovery movement as we now know it started with the publication of first-person accounts of mental health problems in US journals in the 1980s and 1990s (Roberts & Wolfson, 2004; Turner-Crowson & Wallcraft, 2002). These narratives set out how the authors had, by different routes, overcome their difficulties and found satisfying and contributing lives, despite some continuing problems. A number of these papers were written by practitioners with mental health problems (for example, Houghton, 1982; Deegan, 1988; Leete, 1988), some of whom had trained, or taken professional roles, in the context of recovery from long-standing mental health problems. Access to publication and dissemination of ideas was critically important to a new movement that wanted a transfer of power to the powerless. This was facilitated by the willingness of a few scientific journals to publish the personal testimony of service users.

Box 3 sets out some of the themes found in the Recovery literature. It is loosely based on the ideas in Turner-Crowson and Wallcraft's paper of 2002. Our list is neither authoritative nor comprehensive, but is intended to capture the main tenets of the concept of Recovery. One of the first psychiatrists to take a serious academic interest in Recovery was William Anthony at the Rehabilitation Research and Training Centre of Boston University. Twenty years ago, he defined Recovery thus:

Recovery is described as a deeply personal, unique process of changing one's attitudes, values, feelings, goals, skills, and/or roles. It is a way of living a satisfying, hopeful, and contributing life even with limitations caused by illness. Recovery involves the development of new meaning and purpose in one's life as one grows beyond the catastrophic effects of mental illness. Recovery from mental illness involves much more than recovery from the illness itself. People with mental illness may have to recover from the stigma they have incorporated into their very being; from the iatrogenic effects of treatment settings; from lack of recent opportunities for self-determination; from the negative side effects of unemployment; and from crushed dreams. Recovery is often a complex, time-consuming process. (Anthony, 1993, page 527)

> **Box 3** Some themes from the Recovery literature
>
> - *The importance of hope*; the possibility of life beyond medication and illness
> - *Being believed and encouraged*; by at least one person who believes that Recovery is a realistic possibility
> - *Developing perspectives on the past;* grieving what has been lost
> - *Taking personal responsibility for one's life;* making decisions and owning the consequences; managing one's own well-being
> - *Acting to rebuild one's life;* using small steps to avoid failure experiences
> - *Developing valued relationships and roles;* building networks of reciprocal support
> - *Changing expectations of others;* demonstrating capability
> - *Gaining a sense of greater well-being;* aiming for contentment
> - *Developing new meaning and purpose;* which for some includes a spiritual dimension
> - *Persevering;* recognising that set-backs are inevitable and that Recovery is not a linear progression

Some of these ideas had been around for a long time. De-institutionalisation had spawned the development of therapeutic communities. There were local services at Littlemore Hospital, Oxford and in Dingleton Hospital, Melrose (Mandelbrote, 1965; Morrice, 1966) that based local district services around therapeutic communities and adhered to some of the values that are now evident in the Recovery movement. Alcoholics Anonymous was formed in 1935. The organisation developed the idea that Recovery is a life-long process that depends upon people accepting help to take control of their own lives. Franco Basaglia was an Italian psychiatrist who in the 1970s led a left-wing movement for the liberation of people in the psychiatric system, called *Psichiatria Democratica*. The Italian experience demonstrated that radical ideas about mental health care could become national policy in an advanced economy. *Psichiatria Democratica* successfully campaigned for Law 180. This was enacted in 1978 and effectively led to the closure of long-stay mental hospitals in Italy, driving the development of new types of community services. The degree to which this was successful is controversial (e.g. Altamura & Goodwin, 2010; Davidson *et al.*, 2010).

In addition to drawing together existing threads from radical ideas about mental health care, there were some new influences on the Recovery movement. Marius Romme is a Dutch professor of social psychiatry who founded the Hearing Voices movement (Romme & Escher, 1989). He has published work that suggests that hearing voices is not necessarily indicative of mental illness, and that some people who hear voices find the experiences comforting or even pleasurable. Romme regards hearing voices as an understandable reaction to trauma, based upon the type of evidence cited in Chapter 7. The Hearing Voices movement has worked to develop alternatives to drug treatments for distressing voices, in the form of a variety of behavioural and psychological strategies. These include simply accepting that it is OK to hear voices. Related to this has been the emergence of a radical Survivors (of psychiatry) movement. One tendency within the Survivors movement demands the right to be different from other people and to be understood as 'mad' meaning 'righteously angry' rather than 'mad' meaning 'crazy'.

The advance of civil rights activism has resulted in anti-discrimination and disability legislation in many countries. Sections of the community who were shunned and marginalised a few decades ago have successfully asserted their right to participate in society on an equal basis. Although traditional medical attitudes have not disappeared (indeed, they remain common), they run against the equality *zeitgeist*. Paternalism has become steadily less acceptable in mental health services. It is no longer respectable to argue that people with mental illness don't know what is good for them and that they should be passive recipients of services. Service users have gained confidence in insisting that their voices should be heard. Equally important is the rise of the consumer model of health and social care, which emphasises patient choice and looks to market forces to improve the quality of services. Some authoritative voices from within the service user movement (e.g. Perkins, 2001) forcefully advocate the primacy of service user defined outcomes as the aim of treatment, emphasising the potential of consumer choice as a tool to transfer power from professionals to patients.

Does everyone recover?

The Victorian asylums were built in a spirit of therapeutic optimism but they closed with a well-earned reputation as anti-therapeutic warehouses for people with chronic mental illness. One of the major achievements of the Recovery movement has been to confront the mental health professions with their implicit therapeutic nihilism. There is ample evidence that services have encouraged dependency, and in doing so have propagated the idea that treatment should follow a maintenance strategy aimed at keeping at bay an ever-present risk of relapse. Very few clinicians would willingly admit to being negative about the prospect of their patients with psychosis ever getting better, but actions have spoken louder than words. Many psychiatrists continued to follow up patients for decades in the belief that six-monthly appointments were essential to their continued mental stability, or in order to provide emergency back-up, should the need arise.

Although the Recovery movement is primarily based on a set of specific values, there is also an evidence base that lends it support. One element of this evidence is findings from long-term studies of the outcome of psychotic illness. This type of research is difficult to conduct and studies are prone to methodological flaws. Nonetheless, as increasingly reliable findings have become available they have challenged some ideas about the prognosis of psychosis. For example, the International Study of Schizophrenia (ISoS) was an international multicentre study co-ordinated by the World Health Organization (Hopper *et al.*, 2007). Findings were published in 2001 (Harrison *et al.*, 2001b) that suggested that over 50% of people diagnosed with schizophrenia recover eventually, permanently living at home with no psychotic symptoms. Although the early course of the disorder predicted longer-term outcome to some extent, some people experienced late recoveries despite a poor response to treatment early on. There were differences in outcomes between centres, which led the authors to suggest that socio-cultural factors had an important impact. However, 15% of the cohort was still in hospital after 15 to 25 years. Although the modern evidence shows that for most people the outcome of schizophrenia is much better than was previously supposed, there remains an important minority whose problems persist.

There was no golden age of care for people with severe and persistent psychotic symptoms. There has been a long-term tendency for them to be removed from ordinary social settings and forgotten. In the UK they are cared for through 'Out Of Area Placements', meaning that they are placed in private-sector facilities, remote from their families and friends. There have been studies of the care that they receive. Although the living environment in British private-sector psychiatric units is generally better than that offered by equivalent NHS facilities, many aspects of care and treatment appear to be poor. For example, one study examined the care of all patients from a district in the UK who had been placed out of area into eleven different non-forensic private hospitals (Ryan *et al.*, 2004). This showed that almost 80% were locked in, though not legally detained; over 60% had had no multidisciplinary review of their care; there was very little involvement of patients or families in care planning; in 50% of case notes, no comprehensive case history was available; and over a quarter could have been more appropriately cared for in supported accommodation and did not need hospital care at all. The authors commented that '*some patients presented as isolated, vulnerable and powerless to affect their own situations*'. These data were collected three years after the UK Government adopted the Recovery model (Department of Health, 2001). More recent studies have shown a similar picture (e.g. Ryan *et al.*, 2007) and the welfare of this group of people within a changing British health care system·continues to cause serious concern (Killaspy & Meier, 2010).

It would be harsh to judge the implementation of the Recovery model, or indeed any government policy, on the basis that there are still problems in the care of the most disadvantaged people with a mental illness diagnosis. Change takes time. Recovery has challenged the mental health professions to examine deep-seated attitudes and practices that have overemphasised the importance of suppressing symptoms and controlling people, whilst underemphasising the importance of improvements in everyday life. The new assertiveness of the service user movement is an important stage along the way to a different relationship with service providers. However, there is still some cause for concern over the difference between the use of Recovery as a constructive way of challenging professionals to change their practice, and the use of Recovery as a doctrine deployed by health and social service planners.

Mainland Britain hasn't had a revolution since the Civil War of the seventeenth century. It is our cultural tradition to disarm troublesome domestic rebels by assimilating them into the Establishment. It is arguable that the value of the

Recovery idea lies in the tension between its imperatives and the explicit objectives of health policy and practice. Once Recovery has become a key element of policy, its transformative power is disarmed and the way is opened for its use as a euphemism. For example, it is one thing to help people to overcome dependency. It is quite another to offer them no help on the basis that finding your own way promotes Recovery. The same Department of Health document that embraced the Recovery agenda also announced an increased emphasis on safety and a revision of the Mental Health Act that eventually had a negative effect on the freedom and autonomy of people with mental illness (Burns *et al.*, 2013). Herein lies the problem with Recovery. It has an entirely different complexion in the hands of policy makers.

The Inverse Care Law

Julian Tudor Hart is an eminent and radical Welsh general practitioner whose enduring legacy is the Inverse Care Law. He first described this in the *Lancet* in 1971 (Tudor Hart, 1971). The paper is a classic, with 694 citations according to the Web of Science.[2] Tudor Hart best summarised the law:

The availability of good medical care tends to vary inversely with the need for the population served. This inverse care law operates more completely where medical care is most exposed to market forces, and less so where such exposure is reduced. (Tudor Hart, 1971, page 405)

The essential proposition is that the most disadvantaged people have the greatest health need but the worst services.

People with long-term mental health problems caught in the virtual asylum are disadvantaged in securing good-quality services. In their current situation, within well-furnished and freshly decorated total institutions, they have no economic power and few resources to articulate their wishes. They are at the back of the queue for advocacy services. They are the Wrong Kind of Patient owing to their recalcitrance in failing to get better, improvement being implicitly regarded by services as amongst the most important responsibilities of the conscientious patient.

People with mental illnesses that don't improve are likely to have significant problems in their lives that long pre-date the development of psychotic symptoms. There are surprisingly few modern studies of the impact of pre-morbid social factors on outcome in chronic psychosis. Most studies instead investigate poor pre-morbid social functioning, which is taken to be a prodromal symptom of psychosis. However, there is some relevant evidence. Data from the UK700 trial of Psychiatric Assertive Community Treatment were used to assess the effect of occupational and socio-economic status on clinical outcomes (Samele *et al.*, 2001). This showed that the people with the highest best-ever occupational level experienced the best outcomes from psychosis. Highest educational level did not predict

[2] Retrieved 26 April 2013.

outcome. Patients with higher pre-morbid socio-economic status had better outcomes. Downward drift in occupational status did not result in poorer outcomes. This suggests that social factors have a similar impact on outcome to the influence they exert on the risk of developing psychosis in the first place. Immediate social circumstances have less impact than the person's social origins.

In a health system that increasingly looks to market mechanisms to ensure that people with mental illness secure the services that they need, there must be serious concern that people with enduring problems are at a double disadvantage. Both their present circumstances and their social background tend to militate against an equitable and appropriate deployment of health and social care resources. A model of services that takes as its exemplar the educated, articulate person with bipolar affective disorder and places them in control of their treatment through choices over psychological, social and pharmaceutical interventions is entirely appropriate for that type of patient and is likely to work well for them. It is argued by policy makers that the model is just as appropriate for a person with chronic psychosis. The trouble is that this involves a denial of the impact of multiple difficulties, such as isolation from family and friends, restricted personal resources and intrusive psychotic symptoms. Even with professional advocacy support, people in this situation may well find the new health system more difficult to negotiate than the traditional mental health care system. It is not entirely surprising to find that after a decade of the Recovery model, it has yet to make a significant and positive impact within the virtual asylum.

It seems that it may not be sufficient to understand psychotic illness as a catastrophe that hits people at random. For many people diagnosed with psychosis, it is one of a number of problems with a common origin in the circumstances of their childhood. Recovery cannot simply be a matter of being given the power to negotiate the most appropriate package of support and intervention as an informed consumer. Even where this is possible for people with chronic psychosis, simple restoration of one's life to status quo ante might not be an appropriate objective for a large proportion of people for whom the status quo ante was highly unsatisfactory. One critic has pointed to a lack of social context in the founding narratives of the Recovery movement:

Race, gender and class tend to fade away into unexamined background realities, underscoring (intentionally? inadvertently?) the defining centrality of psychiatric disability in these lives. Material deprivation is largely ignored, though poverty and shabby housing bulk large in the lives of many persons with severe mental illness. (Hopper, 2007, page 872)

Is the ghetto such a bad place to be?

It is sometimes said that de-institutionalisation programmes took people with long-term mental health problems and dumped them in flats with financial support but little practical help. The rest of the community had no preparation for their arrival and was either indifferent to their fate or positively hostile to their presence. They were driven into a deep dependency on professional services provided by the state in order to maintain a precarious and unhappy existence outside of the institution. There is a modern concern that largely unreconstructed services are labelling themselves 'Recovery orientated' whilst doing something similar to people newly diagnosed as suffering from psychosis. People are assessed, medicated, CBTed and rehoused, whereupon all support is withdrawn because the state has decided that support is bad for you. Far from promoting Recovery, this is a recipe for social exclusion, because people who were on the margins before they came into contact with services are highly unlikely to find their own way into the mainstream of life.

We saw in Chapter 1 that the risk of schizophrenia associated with growing up in the UK as a person from an African-Caribbean family is reduced where there is a greater density of people from the same ethnic background living in the area (Kirkbride *et al.*, 2007). Although ghettos are defensive formations, necessary in the face of hostility from the rest of the population, there are some advantages to living there.

Richard Warner is a radical British psychiatrist who has worked for many years in Boulder, Colorado. He has impeccable credentials within the Recovery movement. He has lately started to draw attention to the fact that mainstreaming (also known as 'normalisation' or 'social inclusion') isn't necessarily the best route into the community from the margins (Mandiberg & Warner, 2013). He makes a comparison with recent migrants, who do not look to state-sponsored programmes to integrate into indigenous communities. Instead, they form enclave communities, united by identity, which are usually, but not invariably, geographically distinct within a city. These communities develop their own economies and social structures. They eventually become sufficiently successful that they cannot be ignored by the wider community. Integration then happens organically.

The deaf community presents a model of an identity community that has grown in confidence and that has rejected normalisation. Thirty years ago, deaf children were discouraged from using British Sign Language and encouraged to speak and to lip-read. The rationale was that this would allow deaf people to function better in a hearing world. There has been a strong reaction against this, and the deaf community is increasingly assertive that they are a linguistic minority and that British Sign Language is the language of their community. They increasingly refuse to conceptualise hearing impairment as a disability. Disability, they argue, arises from the attitudes of a society that doesn't accommodate to diversity. Some deaf people choose to live mainly within the deaf community, others live partially within it, and some deaf people choose not to be part of it. The deaf community is self-defining and it creatively facilitates people's lives on the terms that they choose.

Warner argues that these models are applicable to people with serious mental illness. He acknowledges that there are no thriving identity communities of people with mental illness at present, but he does cite some examples of projects that have some of the necessary characteristics, for example clustered housing schemes that are managed by the residents, and the clubhouse movement in the USA. Warner sees a way forward towards integration through social businesses by and for people with mental illness diagnoses. External help takes the form of business incubators, focussed on overcoming obstructions to business development such as access to capital for a group of people who tend to have poor credit histories. This might allow, for example, the establishment of co-operative pharmacies for and by people with mental health problems, recycling money back into the identity community, cash that would otherwise disappear into big business. Many mental health services already employ service users and there is no reason why the free-standing social enterprise model should not work.

The emphasis on collective action, on people with mental illness diagnoses setting their own objectives as a community and collectively taking control of services to meet their needs, is highly attractive. It is compatible with taking social context into account rather than focussing solely upon mental illness diagnoses. It creates a model of Recovery that is based on more than simple consumer choices.

Recovery versus safety

One of the things that makes mental health services a continuous source of controversy is the issue of safety. It is objectively true that people with mental health problems are at risk of harming themselves and that there is a very small but distinct risk of harming other people. People with mental health problems sometimes behave in unusual and unpredictable ways that create hazards for themselves and others, independent of any intention to cause harm.

There is a cogent argument that Recovery and safety are not in conflict with each other (Davidson *et al.*, 2006). Who would want to be unsafe? Being safe and secure is one of the elements of Recovery. However, it is with respect to safety that the largest gap appears between Recovery as an objective of people with mental illness diagnoses, and Recovery as a model for policy makers. For the latter, safety and control are indivisible. The only advantage of inpatient settings as therapeutic environments is the degree of control over patients that they offer (Poole & Higgo, 2008), and it is here that expectations of safety are greatest. Control, however, is very hard to square with a Recovery orientation. There have been efforts to devise models that somehow reconcile the conflict between the two imperatives (for example, Roychowdhury, 2011). These are partial solutions at best, whereby paternalism takes precedence in matters central to risk, and Recovery principles apply to everything else.

The use of compulsion

The problem is that it isn't possible to take partial personal responsibility for yourself. If you have the right to decide for yourself but your choices are limited to good decisions, then you have no autonomy at all. Alongside UK policy makers' attachment to an ill-defined form of the Recovery model, there has been unrelenting emphasis on detention and legal control. In 2007, the Mental Health Act for England and Wales was amended. The big change was the introduction of Community Treatment Orders (CTOs), a form of long-term compulsory treatment in the community. Organised psychiatry, including the Royal College of Psychiatrists, fought hard alongside other mental health organisations in a principled struggle to stop CTOs being introduced, on the basis that they involve unnecessary restrictions to the autonomy of people with mental illness. Once CTOs were introduced, however, the same group of doctors that had resisted their introduction used them in far larger numbers than had ever been anticipated (Lepping & Malik, 2013). There is evidence that CTOs are being widely used to contain risk, when the intention was that they should be used to prevent relapse. A well-conducted randomised controlled trial of CTOs, the OCTET study, has recently been reported (Burns et al., 2013). It has convincingly shown that, when used in the UK, CTOs have no benefits for patients over previous practice. There are no advantages in the use of CTOs to offset the deprivation of freedom that they entail. The OCTET research group argue that the evidence is so convincing that it is now unethical to use CTOs. It is too soon to know whether the profession will take heed of this, but it seems unlikely. Psychiatrists had serious misgivings about CTOs before they were ever introduced, but this has not prevented their widespread use.

In addition to new forms of legal compulsion on people with mental illness, the existing powers to detain are being used increasingly frequently. In 2011–12, the number of people subject to a CTO in England increased by 11%, but the number detained in hospital increased by 5% (Health and Social Care Information Centre, Community and Mental Health Team, 2012). These were part of long-term trends. The number of people detained in independent-sector hospitals rose by 21%. There is no convoluted logic that can make these figures consistent with a national policy of Recovery-orientated services. In the absence of any evidence of a national epidemic of serious mental illness, it is clear that we are increasingly imposing formal controls on people diagnosed with mental illness.

It is possible that services for the majority of service users have become more Recovery-orientated and user-friendly whilst a high-risk minority are being exposed to an entirely different service philosophy. This seems extremely unlikely. The awareness that services are progressively lowering their threshold for compulsory intervention is bound to have a significant impact on a much larger number of people than ever experience compulsory treatment. This awareness probably undermines therapeutic alliances between psychiatrists and their patients in general.

The burden of increased compulsion falls disproportionately upon urban working-class communities. The annual rate of detention in 2011–12 in the London Strategic Health Authority (SHA) area was 80 per 100,000. In the East of England SHA area it was 40 per 100,000. London is the most urban of England's SHA areas, with some areas of severe deprivation. East of England is one of the most rural and prosperous areas of the country. Even if Recovery-orientated services are a reality for some NHS service users, it appears that this is least likely to be the case for the most deprived part of the population. They have the highest risk of developing a major mental illness in the first place and they face the greatest barriers to a good outcome. The Inverse Care Law casts a long shadow over mental health services.

Defensive practice

Organised psychiatry recognised the importance of the Recovery movement relatively quickly, which is laudable in the light of the obvious threat to the profession's status that is intrinsic to some Recovery ideas. The profession continues to make firm statements in support of Recovery's conceptual framework (for example, South London and Maudsley NHS Foundation Trust and South West and St George's Mental Health NHS Trust, 2010). There is a paradox in the contradictions in British psychiatry's attitudes to CTOs; as noted above, once the fight over their introduction was lost, psychiatrists embraced their use with gusto. The committed anti-psychiatric lobby may feel that this shows that the profession's liberal sentiments have shallow roots compared with a more deep-seated need to have personal control over patients. However, this type of individual psychological explanation has very limited explanatory power, as it begs the question as to why psychiatrists should have a need to exert control over patients in the first place.

As mentioned in Chapter 8, there is a great deal of rhetoric within mental health services about the need for creative risk taking in the care of people with mental health problems. There is also much discussion about the need for a no-blame culture within organisations so that professionals can be frank and learn lessons when things go wrong; about the statistical inevitability of occasional tragedies such as suicide or homicide in services that have contact with very large numbers of people every year; and about the difference between predictability and preventability of untoward incidents. None of this rhetoric has any positive impact on professional behaviour. We live in the era of anxious practice and there is absolutely no evidence of any reduction in risk aversion. This is due to a widespread awareness that when things go wrong there is no such thing as a no-blame culture. Serious untoward incidents are followed by internal investigations, police involvement, external inquiries, coroners' inquests, trial by media and medical litigation. It is unusual for mental health professionals to be sacked, demoted or disciplined as a direct result. Amongst all the professions, it is especially unusual for psychiatrists to suffer such consequences. However, it is not the outcome of investigations that clinicians find intimidating. It is the process that causes fear.

Most clinicians are distressed and self-reproachful when things go wrong, even where objectively speaking there is little they could have done to prevent the incident. The various processes cause damage to their self-esteem and to their reputation. Most psychiatrists have seen colleagues go through these ordeals, which can last for a year or more. The policy contradictions between risk and Recovery can transform well-meaning, Recovery-orientated psychiatrists into over-cautious authoritarians, because the alternative is too anxiety-provoking. When making plans for patients who they perceive to be at risk, psychiatrists routinely consider how they might answer the question 'Why did you choose not to apply for a CTO?' from an imagined inquisitor.

The underlying preoccupations of mental health services remain focussed on compliance and symptom resolution rather than quality of life as defined by patients. In claiming to be Recovery-orientated, the language of Recovery is bound to be distorted into euphemisms for professional attitudes and practices that are based on a completely different set of values. As David Pilgrim has written:

Coercive policing from one perspective is warranted care from another. One perspective's unwanted interference is another's duty of care. One perspective's lack of insight due to impairment and illness is another's suppressed choice and discounted agency. (Pilgrim, 2008, page 300)

Seen from these perspectives, UK mental health policy has an intrinsic lack of consistency and logic. Nonetheless, it is far from clear that making safety a high priority in policy is inappropriate. Mental health professionals are generally positive about their ability to prevent suicide, but non-specialist health professionals are more fatalistic, with scepticism that they can prevent it (Herron et al., 2001). Preventing avoidable death is a primary responsibility of all health professionals. Suicide is a tragedy with long-lasting consequences for families. Homicides, if anything, are worse. Attempting to optimise the safety of patients in contact with mental health services is a reasonable and legitimate objective. There are two questions to be taken into account that somewhat temper this. Firstly, does compulsion enhance safety, or are there other, less intrusive measures that might enhance safety more effectively? Secondly, are safety measures proportionate to risk? In other words is the extent of the loss of freedom justified by the size or nature of the risk? How many people are affected by a loss of freedom to prevent one adverse incident?

Persuasion

Unfortunately, it is difficult to give reliable answers to these questions. The OCTET research (see above) was unusual in the UK literature in randomising participants to two different legal measures. It would be very difficult to get the necessary ethical and other permissions for a randomised trial comparing compulsion with no compulsion. Compulsion in the psychiatric literature is usually taken to mean formal legal measures. There is an emerging literature on other types of pressure that are used to persuade people to accept treatment. This is known as 'leverage'. A recent UK study found that a third of people with psychosis reported having been subject to leverage, compared with two thirds of people with a substance-misuse diagnosis and a sixth of people with a non-psychosis, non-substance misuse diagnosis (Burns et al., 2011). The commonest type of leverage related to accommodation, which affected 20% of those with psychosis and 44% of those with substance-misuse problems. In other words provision of accommodation was conditional on tenants accepting treatment. Other types of leverage included contact with children and conditions imposed by courts. Compared with a similar US study, direct leverage ('accept treatment or go to prison') was less common in the UK, and direct financial leverage ('you won't get your money if you don't accept treatment') was much less common.

Leverage is different from coercion. Whilst it involves exerting pressure on people to conduct themselves in a desired fashion, it can be viewed as confronting people with the inevitable consequences of certain choices. Social landlords have obligations towards all of their tenants, and people who are psychotic can be very troubling neighbours. Life is led in social configurations that are characterised by reciprocation. Individuals who fail to meet accepted minimum standards of reciprocation are generally considered to be criminals or psychopaths. Although neo-classical economists base their theories on the idea that people are 'rational' in so far as they are claimed to be entirely selfish and individualistic, there is ample evidence that this is not the case (Dawnay & Shah, 2005). Theories based on these assumptions failed to predict the global financial catastrophe of 2008. Decisions to neglect your own health have an impact on other people, such as family, friends and neighbours. Society at large has a legitimate interest in public order and the expense involved in providing care and support for people who are mentally ill. Many of the features of mental health services that have been abusive or counter-therapeutic can be regarded as abuses of human rights. The need to avoid human rights violations does not imply that the interest of society in individuals' mental health is not legitimate. Instead, it means that the imperatives of society at large have to be balanced with individual rights.

In some ways, leverage is a good thing. The high level of leverage experienced by people in substance-misuse services is probably due to partners threatening to end relationships unless people get help with their substance-misuse problem. This is entirely reasonable, and it is a factor that is known to be associated with stabilisation and abstinence. When people with mental illness have recovered after accepting help under interpersonal duress of this sort, they often acknowledge that leverage was helpful though they disliked it at the time.

Let's rename the Recovery Star

Recovery has become so reified that we now have a Recovery psychometric instrument, the Recovery Star. Enthusiasts claim that it measures a single underlying Recovery construct so that the degree of Recovery can be measured objectively (Dickens et al., 2012). However, the Recovery Star has a marked resemblance to many previous instruments that have been used within rehabilitation services for decades to track progress of people with complex problems. Attempts to objectively measure an intrinsically subjective perception such as Recovery is illogical, and in any case there are doubts over the Recovery Star's psychometric properties as a measure of change.[3] Whilst there is no doubt that the instrument is useful, its connection to Recovery per se is dubious. It stands as a concrete metaphor for the expropriation of Recovery terminology by professionals.

So it is for so-called Recovery-orientated services. Statutory mental health services can play an important role in Recovery, though people can recover without them. What services cannot do is follow a consistent Recovery model for all patients at all times, because services are subject to legitimate imperatives that contradict fundament aspects of the Recovery model. Sometimes, the Recovery model simply isn't appropriate or possible. Some people, under some circumstances, need someone to tell them what to do, because they are simply incapable of making decisions for themselves. This is not incompatible with recovery. It should be remembered that the participants in the ISoS study, which showed a better than expected outcome of schizophrenia, were not treated in Recovery-orientated services. The majority were treated within old-fashioned institutional psychiatry with all its undoubted faults, and they still recovered in the majority of cases.

Failure to recognise that services sometimes need to be controlling would lead us to a Szaszian nightmare where seriously ill people who lacked mental capacity would face punitive consequences of behaviour driven by psychosis. 'Recovery-orientated' is a poor, euphemistic term that is seriously misleading. Recovery belongs to people with mental illness, not to professionals.

Collectivism versus individualism

It is discomforting to point out that a number of elements of the Recovery model have a strong resonance for governments that adhere to neo-liberal economic policies. One is an emphasis on personal choice, which points to a market-driven model of mental health care with multiple providers and price competition. Another is the rejection of dependency on services, suggesting early disengagement and limitations on costs.

It is far from clear that the British population attaches much importance to the ability to choose between health care providers. Research consistently shows that people want good-quality local services that can be accessed in a timely way (Coulter, 2005). Amongst the features of good-quality services, it is human qualities of practitioners that are most highly rated. These are regarded as considerably more important than technical excellence. Mental health service users value trustworthiness in clinicians, and they want to be involved in decisions (Laugharne & Priebe, 2006). It is far from clear that choice of provider organisation is even regarded as relevant by patients.

[3] Killaspy H, Boardman J, King M *et al*. The Mental Health Recovery Star: great for care planning but not as a routine outcome measure. *The Psychiatrist eletter* published online 21 February 2012 *retrieved 12 May 2013*.

The type of coercion and control that was prevalent in the asylums of the past was anti-therapeutic and an affront to humanitarian values. We have developed new coercive measures, and the issue of control shows no sign of disappearing. There are other ways forward, if we choose to take them. Psychiatrists will probably always have to deploy leverage in a skilled and ethical way, and this is always going to create tensions in therapeutic relationships that have to be managed by doctor and patient alike. Mental health services in the inner cities need to have the capability to work with the consequences of multiple deprivations and they must be well-resourced, because demand is high. There are some really fine inner-city services in the UK, but there are some poor ones too. As our health services change, it is going to be important to remember about the Inverse Care Law. There are few more radical objectives in mental health care than the provision of really high-quality services in the inner cities.

Main points in this chapter

1. The Recovery model has been an important development in the service user movement that has challenged professionals to change their practice.
2. It is not a panacea. The branding of the entire government programme of mental health legislation and provision as 'Recovery-orientated' is a policy oxymoron, which is misleading and helpful.
3. The state-sponsored version of the Recovery model is sometimes used as a rationale to promote market models of health care and to minimise or withdraw services.
4. The Recovery model is not always the most appropriate model for the most vulnerable and unwell people. To pretend otherwise does not serve them well.
5. The Recovery model has a core message of hope that is its greatest strength.

10

Working with poverty

To recap, the intimate relationship between poverty and serious mental health problems has a number of consequences for clinical practice. The prevalence of psychosis is much higher in deprived inner-city areas. Wherever they are located, mental health services are predominantly utilised by people from the poorest section of the community. Even in wealthier areas, the majority of service users come from a poorer local minority. In general, poverty makes it more difficult to recover from mental health problems, so poor people tend to experience severe illnesses and to stay in services longer. As a wide range of different social and health problems are strongly associated with poverty and particularly inner-city deprivation, a high proportion of service users have multiple and complex problems. These difficulties have common origins. Mental health professionals in the UK spend most of their time treating people with lifelong experience of poverty. Even the private sector in this country predominantly provides services for poor people.

Modern social psychiatry

Social psychiatry was the dominant approach in British psychiatric research for several decades after the Second World War. UK psychiatric researchers are world leaders in investigating the interaction between social, genetic and developmental factors in causing mental disorders. It is only recently that psychiatric research has begun to adopt models of poverty, social class and urbanicity that have any degree of sophistication. There was a time towards the end of the twentieth century when there was optimism (ill-founded, as it turned out) that relatively straightforward explanations of the causation of major mental disorders would be found through molecular genetics. During that period it felt as if social inequalities were being treated as simple confounding factors that obstructed a proper understanding of biological processes, rather than as complex elements of people's lives that powerfully shape behaviour and disorder through interaction with genetic and other influences.

Mental illnesses happen in people's lives. An illness, mental or otherwise, that makes no difference to the things that someone does or to their interactions with other people could hardly be regarded as an illness at all (here we will resist the temptation to explore interesting questions such as whether mild to moderate hypertension can be regarded as an illness, a disease or neither). Whilst the precise causes of mental illness remain obscure, we know that housing, employment, social networks, culture and education all have an effect on its incidence, and just as much effect on the likelihood of true recovery. The twenty-first century has seen psychiatry emerge from a long period of neglect of its social aspects.

As evidence has accumulated that social environment has a central importance in psychiatry, both scientifically and clinically, there has been a major upsurge in interest in social factors evident in general psychiatry journals and in the form of new books. Whilst it is clear that a type of clinical practice that engages with the social environment is the most appropriate way of working with people in deprivation, what we do not have is a clear and generally accepted model of what modern social psychiatry really is. It has been repeatedly claimed that social psychiatry is difficult to define. Twenty years ago a British textbook of social psychiatry stated: *'The simplest definition of social psychiatry is that it is what is done by social psychiatrists'* (Bhugra & Leff, 1993, page 3). This kind of tautological definition is unhelpful, especially as there is a core of continuing themes that link social psychiatry traditions of the past and present. As an intellectual tradition, social psychiatry is as distinctive as biological psychiatry or cognitive behavioural psychotherapy. It has particular utility in addressing the complex clinical problems that arise in working with deprived populations.

No matter what 'social psychiatry' may have meant in the past, the main themes in modern social psychiatry include the following:

- Social psychiatry takes as its primary focus the way that people live and interact with each other, and the impact that this has on their mental health. It is concerned with meaningful contexts and factors that can be seen, experienced and altered.
- Social psychiatry draws upon both the macroscopic behaviours of populations (for example, through epidemiology or an understanding of culture) and the study of individual behaviour (for example, in understanding the origins and effects of patterns of emotional expression in families, or the protective nature of networks of support).
- Social psychiatry does not reject the importance of psychological or biological factors. It does not necessarily look for 'ultimate' causations in social factors. One of its strengths is that it can have utility whilst remaining relatively atheoretical.
- Social psychiatry cannot ignore issues of culture and meaning, because all human behaviour is affected by them. It is necessary to acknowledge the importance of

values, which affect the approach to difficult issues such as ethnicity and racism. Practitioners have to be clear about their own values.

- Social psychiatry is the clinical orientation that is most closely concerned with everyday meaning. With a focus on tangible realities, social psychiatry draws clinicians towards a type of clinical practice that can be experienced by service users as relevant to problems in their lives as they are lived.
- Social psychiatry is particularly helpful in achieving an accommodation between the demands of science (that objectivity should prevail and that measurement, evaluation and replicability are important) without losing contact with the things that are important to patients and their families.
- Social psychiatry does not confine itself to interventions at the individual level. Relationships, families, kinship networks, communities and public health are also arenas for intervention.
- Social psychiatry draws the clinician to practise within the patient's social environment. Seeing patients in their home, rather than in hospital, leads to many other changes in clinical practice. These distinctive ways of working are the foundations of community psychiatry.
- Social psychiatry cannot avoid broad questions of social policy affecting whole populations, such as the effects of social disadvantage. This brings the social psychiatrist into the arena of public health, where change always has a political implication. This unavoidable interaction with the political creates a difficult tension, as scientific credibility can be undermined if one strays into ideological proselytisation.
- Social psychiatry is above all pragmatic. It can be extremely difficult to lift people out of poverty when they have a mental health problem, but it is possible and it is important to try. Helping a patient to resolve a housing problem or to find employment is often more important in overcoming mental illness than achieving optimal drug treatment.

None of this should be taken as an argument for a narrow social focus in psychiatry. Despite the difficulties in scientifically integrating the psychological, the social and the biological, each has to be attended to in clinical practice. Until the necessary paradigm shift occurs, clinicians need ways of thinking about mental disorders that minimise the pitfalls caused by the tensions within the biopsychosocial compromise described in Chapter 7.

Class difference and power gradients

Mental health professionals are well educated and tend to come from less deprived or from comfortable backgrounds. There is a power imbalance between clinicians and patients that is intrinsic to all therapeutic relationships, which is greatly exacerbated by the statutory powers of psychiatrists to detain and control people. A previous book explored some ways of managing this within therapeutic relationships (Poole & Higgo, 2006). There is a further effect arising from class difference. One of the key attributes of human beings is their ability to empathise and to understand people with very different lives to themselves. Without this ability, fiction wouldn't be entertaining, it would just be puzzling. It is not necessary to be similar to someone else to understand them. However, mental health professionals don't always recognise how different their life experience is from that of their patients. Effective mental health professionals have to be able to recognise different lifestyles, and to learn about them, not didactically, but by talking with and listening to patients and families.

Class difference can create a barrier to trust. People from deprived backgrounds occasionally show a deference to authority figures that masks disdain. We pointed out in Chapter 2 that people in deprived communities can have an ambivalent attitude to authority, on the one hand experiencing it as persecutory, but on the other hand feeling let down or neglected. This is not a good basis for a constructive therapeutic relationship, especially where the person is suffering from a psychotic illness. An awareness in the clinician of the nature of the difficulty helps, because few liberal professionals find it easy to see themselves as someone else's untrustworthy authority figure.

Both medicine and nursing have come under sustained attack in recent years, and there have been a number of scandals that might reasonably have been expected to erode public confidence in the professions. In fact, based on opinion-poll findings, this has not happened at all. A large majority of the general public regard doctors and nurses as intrinsically highly trustworthy. 'Doctor' and 'nurse' are not just job descriptions. They are social roles, vessels created by the expectations of others into which individuals are uncomfortably poured. The strength of the expectations attached to the social role 'doctor' is one of the reasons why some are reluctant to admit to their profession to strangers in social gatherings.

Trustworthiness is the key attribute of the social roles of 'doctor' and 'nurse'. Deviant individuals, like Dr Harold Shipman, who are found to have betrayed the trust expectation, are condemned and regarded as monsters. Their personal betrayal of trust doesn't alter the expectation of the behaviour of all other doctors. Who would ever give sensitive information to, or accept potentially hazardous treatments from, strangers who they didn't trust? The perception of trustworthiness is an absolute necessity if people are to accept health care at all.

The expectation of trustworthiness may not be held as strongly by people who are highly marginalised. Some people diagnosed as having personality disorder come to be very suspicious of health professionals, on the basis of their experience of services rather than their background characteristics. It is by no means impossible to engage and work constructively with people under these circumstances, but, inconveniently, trust must be earned. Building trust is an active task that must be given attention. For the most part this means avoiding being patronising, being clear and honest, and avoiding doing or saying difficult things in such a way as might be experienced as undermining whatever fragile trust has been established. Most of all, it is necessary to remember that, no matter how friendly your relationship with the patient and their family, it is being conducted across a steep power gradient. This issue does not disappear, even after lengthy contact.

Care pathways

We have examined the shortcomings of care pathways in mental health elsewhere (Poole & Higgo, 2008). There is a strong movement, driven in part by concerns over quality of care, driven in part by economic considerations, to develop standardised programmes of care for people with specific diagnoses. Irrespective of the supposed advantages for people with uncomplicated mental health problems, care pathways work badly where people have multiple or complex difficulties. They find themselves on more than one care pathway (usually sequentially) or they find themselves suitable for no care pathway. Working with poverty means that services have to assume that a very high proportion (usually the majority) of people with mental health problems will have complex difficulties. There are claims that complex problems can be adequately managed through multiple specialist teams (Rosen *et al.*, 2013), but we are more sympathetic to claims that genericism, being highly flexible, is the model that works best under most circumstances.[1]

In Chapters 6 and 9 we discussed the tendency of people from deprived communities and with complex problems to be regarded as the Wrong Kind of Patient. Care pathways are a type of Fordism applied to health care. They are predicated on the belief that uniform processes can be quality controlled to create predictable outcomes. There is a political aspiration to create discrete packages of care that can be managed as products within health-care markets. This may work well for people for whom a mental health problem is a relatively encapsulated difficulty. The trouble is that even where the patient comes from a comfortable background, this encapsulation is likely to be more apparent than real. Life is messy and complicated, and effective mental health services have to be able to respond to this. The Wrong Kind of Patient is identified as such by the services because their multiple problems interact with each other in such a way that it is impossible to pretend that they neatly fit into a single specialist service or care pathway.

In order to meet the needs of people living in poverty and who face multiple problems, services have to be flexible and need to develop ways of working that suit local populations. Rigid programmes of care will fail for a significant proportion of people with heterogeneous difficulties. People need to be able to access effective components of care that meet their actual needs without conforming to arbitrary criteria that meet the organisational needs of services.

---

[1] Burns T. Newer is not automatically better. *The Psychiatrist* eletter published on-line 22 October 2012 pb.rcpsych.org/content/36/10/361/reply#pbrcpsych_el_18266 *retrieved 5 November 2012.*

To take an example, most psychiatric inpatient units strongly resist admitting people who are intoxicated with alcohol and who say that they want to kill themselves. If admitted, a very high proportion of people like this will be sober the next day and will display no further intention of harming themselves. There is usually little or no benefit from admissions like this. They are a poor use of scarce inpatient resources. However, there is a group of people who have a primary alcohol problem who repeatedly make serious suicide attempts when drunk in the absence of a continuing suicidal intention when sober. This can follow an escalating pattern. It can become obvious to family and friends that unless someone intervenes to address their drinking whilst simultaneously ensuring their safety, they will eventually kill themselves. Substance-misuse services find it hard to respond, because they are not organised to make emergency interventions. Psychiatric services exclude them because they have a substance-misuse problem and they are not mentally ill. They are the Wrong Kind of Patients, and some of them die as a consequence. Emergency admission and detoxification can lead to long-term abstinence if followed through properly. The intervention is potentially life-saving. There are other similar scenarios, and they are by no means rare. Perusal of the serious untoward incident reports that are produced by mental health services when things go wrong suggests that a large proportion of incidents involve people who are the Wrong Kind of Patient. It is an indictment of services that we have potentially effective interventions that we choose not to deploy with certain types of patient because they do not meet criteria or the intervention doesn't fit in with the preferred pattern of service provision. This can be put right, but only if there is a political and professional will to do so.

Narrative as an integrative framework

Although it is possible to understand people's problems by having separate biological, psychological and social formulations, this is clumsy. It doesn't create a representation of the person that is very realistic or meaningful. The biological, the psychological and the social are only separate because of human limitations in understanding complexity. Out there in the world, they are parts of an existence that is unitary. The key device that we have found useful in holding together biological, psychological and social factors in a coherent and balanced way has been a particular application of narrative to clinical problems.

The use of narrative has attracted a good deal of attention in recent years as a qualitative method of exploring subjective patient experience of disease and health care. This has intrinsic value. However, narrative can also serve an empirical function in psychiatry. There is nothing new in this assertion. Throughout the English-speaking world, it was long taken as a truism that careful history taking was the cornerstone of sound clinical practice. In the UK, two influences emphasised the importance of placing psychopathology in a meaningful context. The first was the tradition of meticulous and detailed history-taking that was passed down the generations through the enduring popularity of the *Maudsley Handbook of*

Practical Psychiatry (Murray & Goldberg, 2006), which is the descendant of a small booklet known as 'The Orange Book'. The emphasis on this approach was largely due to the influence of Sir Aubrey Lewis, professor of psychiatry at the Institute of Psychiatry from 1946 to 1966. As a young psychiatrist Lewis had worked with Adolph Meyer and was impressed by his ideas. Lewis was a shy, brilliant man who inspired and terrified an entire generation of British academic psychiatrists. British psychiatry still bears his mark, 50 years after his retirement.

The other influence was the approach to understanding psychopathology that was developed by Karl Jaspers and other German-speaking phenomenologists. This influence arrived with refugee psychiatrists fleeing the Nazis, but it was spread in the UK through Frank Fish's seminal books (Fish, 1967; Hamilton, 1984). The approach emphasises the importance of the psychological context in which abnormalities arise, and requires the psychiatrist to consciously develop empathy for the patient's frame of mind in order to understand what is going on.

Prominent amongst the advances in psychiatry in recent decades has been more reliable and consistent diagnosis, reflected in the development of successive editions of the American Psychiatric Association's Diagnostic and Statistical Manual (DSM) and the International Classification of Disease (ICD). There have also been advances in the training of psychiatrists.

All advances have drawbacks, and there is a widespread perception that the new nosological systems have led to an overemphasis on diagnosis as an all-embracing way of understanding mental health problems. At the time of writing the fifth edition of DSM, DSM-V, is about to be published amid great controversy, as it is widely believed to have parted company with the scientific evidence. Indeed, it appears that the entire American consensus on nosology may now unravel. The US National Institute of Mental Health have announced that they do not intend to use DSM-V, hoping instead for a classification based on neuroscience and genetics. To British psychiatrists, this is at best premature, at worst fanciful.

Training under the old apprenticeship system was excellent if you happened to work with good trainers, but it was very unsatisfactory if you did not. Modern training has achieved greater consistency by becoming more programmatic and procedural. Similar to the sense that manualised diagnosis has become reified and is now a problem, proceduralised training has, in some hands, neglected the acquisition of skills, reducing history-taking to a checklist of demographic details. Mental-state examination has been vulgarised into a record of what patients say rather than what they experience.

Skilled psychiatrists engage patients in a process of developing a narrative about their illness, which is both empirically accurate and meaningful to the patient. The process allows the psychiatrist to understand the patient's problems with reference to a range of relevant biological, psychological and social factors, which are woven into a single story. Developing a shared narrative has an intrinsic therapeutic value, allowing most patients to move from fear and confusion over their experiences to a contextualised understanding that allows them to see what the way forward might be. Such narratives usually include a diagnosis, and an understanding of what that diagnosis means. The narrative has to have a demonstrable objective truth, with links to tangible facts and events, for it to have any usefulness.

Such narratives rarely arrive completely formed after a single meeting. They develop over time. 'Truth' under these circumstances includes an aspect of personal meaning. The same event, for example a termination of pregnancy, can have different meanings to different people, which might include relief, shame, guilt, indifference and regret (or indeed any combination or sequence of these). This personal and subjective element does not undermine the empirical nature of the narrative. Indeed, different meaning-laden reactions to specific types of events (such as bereavement) have measurable effects, all the way down to their impact on the cellular components of the immune system.

At a more abstract level, years of clinical practice exposes mental health practitioners to hundreds or thousands of narratives. Within these accumulated stories there are repeated patterns and trajectories that represent the common routes by which mental illness arises in people's lives, as opposed to in their brains or in their minds. Scientific understanding and empirical evidence has to be applied to these meta-narratives and to individual narratives. This is the essence of making psychiatry a true applied science.

A narrative

To put some flesh on the process of the development of a narrative, let us take the fictional example of Alan, a 63-year-old man who was taken to the local Accident and Emergency department after the police had spotted him trying to drown himself in a river close to his home. After a night in hospital, he was declared physically fit, and a psychiatrist assessed him. He told the psychiatrist that he had tried to kill himself because he had developed a tremor and he had lost all feelings in his hands. His general practitioner could find no cause for his symptoms, but Alan was certain that he had a degenerative neurological condition. He did not wish to become a burden to his family, and he had come to feel that it would be better for everyone if he was dead. He had put his affairs in order, and waited until he was sure that he would not be disturbed whilst he drowned himself. When this judgement proved incorrect, he co-operated with the police officers' efforts to save him, but he regretted that the attempt had failed. When asked if he might do something similar again, he would only say that the psychiatrist would have to make his own mind up about that.

Naturally, the assessing psychiatrist was concerned about the continuing risk of suicide. He established that Alan lived alone in a house that he had shared with his wife until she had died of cancer three years earlier. He was retired, with a pension from his job as an electrician. His two daughters lived nearby and they were supportive, though they were both busy with young families. Alan denied feeling depressed, but he did admit to being worried about his physical health. However, the psychiatrist found clear evidence of a depressive illness, with sleep disturbance, impaired concentration, weight loss, anhedonia and marked depressive cognitions. He diagnosed major depression associated with a high suicide risk. Alan reluctantly agreed to admission to a psychiatric inpatient unit, where he was started on an antidepressant.

Clinical histories of this nature are common, and the diagnosis and assessment of risk were correct. At this point, Alan's story, as far as he was concerned, was that 'there was nothing down for him'; that everything that gave him pleasure and made life meaningful was in the past and could not be regained; that he was living on limited funds; and that he now had a degenerative disease that no one could identify or treat. On top of everything else, a psychiatrist seemed to think he was mentally ill, when it seemed quite obvious to Alan that his current feelings were an appropriate reaction to his circumstances. There was nothing he could do to improve his situation, and therefore he would be better off dead.

The process of forming a more accurate and constructive narrative that was shared by doctor and patient spanned a number of interviews over several weeks. It was embedded in the psychiatrist trying to understand better what had happened to Alan to bring him to these symptoms at this time. It involved active participation from both doctor and patient. Sometimes it involved the psychiatrist trying to change Alan's understanding of his symptoms, for example, that the numbness and tremor in his hands were directly related to anxiety and hyperventilation, and not to neurological disease. This was assisted by his ability to show that breathing exercises eased the symptoms. Sometimes Alan had to get the psychiatrist to see that he had misunderstood. For example, initially the psychiatrist attributed Alan's depression to unresolved grief over the death of his wife. However, both Alan and his daughters disagreed. They felt that he had grieved normally. Alan's wife had been by far the more sociable of the couple. After she died, Alan was ill-equipped to form a social life, and, having nursed her for a couple of years, he had nothing to do any more. Isolation and loneliness are different to grief and they have different solutions.

Eventually, Alan got better. The narrative that doctor and patient formed did not conflict with the psychiatrist's initial assessment, but it was a more detailed, constructive and true account of Alan's situation. Alan had grown up in children's homes, and he knew virtually nothing about his parents. He had been a solitary, anxious child whose academic performance was poor. He had tended to exist on the fringes of the gangs of children in the homes and in school, neither at the centre of the groupings nor a rejected outcast. At sixteen he had joined the Army. For the first time, he felt secure and functioned well. He trained as an electrician, where his somewhat obsessional perfectionism was an asset.

In his late twenties a girl struck up a conversation with him on a train. Not long after, he left the Army and they married. They went to live close to her parents, and his father-in-law helped him to secure a post as an electrician in the factory where he worked. Alan's wife had a strong Christian faith, and although his own faith was less intense, he attended church with her. Their social life was mainly focussed on her involvement with the church. Their daughters were soon born, and Alan was content with his quiet, settled family life. In his early forties he felt progressively weaker, more tired and more miserable. This was eventually found to be due to tuberculosis, presumed to have been contracted overseas whilst in the Army. His treatment necessitated a lengthy absence from work, and he feared that he might lose his job. He was valued by his employers, and he felt a real sense of gratitude to them when he returned to his old post.

Alan's life drifted on satisfactorily through his middle years, unperturbed by his daughters leaving home and the arrival of grandchildren. In truth, his relationship with his offspring and their children alike was kindly but distant, as he was never really sure how he should be with youngsters.

Things changed in the years running up to his suicide attempt, which were very difficult for him. Firstly, the factory closed, and Alan had no option but to take early retirement on a reduced pension. His wife became ill and died. She had always looked after him, and he now nursed her, which kept him very busy.

Once his wife had gone, he found himself isolated. The church and parishioners tried to be supportive, but, lacking social skills as he did, he felt painfully awkward at their social gatherings without his wife's protective presence. There was work that needed to be carried out on the house, but he was short of money. Instead of getting the work done in stages, he worried, and increasingly checked the safety of the wiring, the plumbing, the gas supply and the drains. As he became more miserable, he found his grandchildren's boisterousness hard to tolerate. He further isolated himself. He tried to comfort himself with binge drinking. His experience of tuberculosis, together with his wife's recent death, made him hypervigilant with respect to his health, so that the physical effects of his growing anxiety fed upon themselves and bred gloomy self-diagnosis. All in all, one could see how he had come to be so dangerously low in mood.

Understood in this way, the narrative offered a guide to potential solutions. For example, there would be little point in trying to overcome his isolation through involvement in the church's social activities, as he would experience this as a stress. However, he could offer his services as a handyman through the church, which would give life some structure and purpose, and enable him to have social contact in a role that was familiar to him.

This narrative draws together a range of biological, psychological and social factors in a coherent way, and it illustrates some of the complex ways in which social disadvantage can play out in someone's life, making them more vulnerable to the development of mental illness. This is not a story of grinding material deprivation, but of persistent ramifications of early disadvantage. To draw out just a few themes:

- As mentioned in Chapter 7, children who grow up in institutional care are one of the most disadvantaged populations in Western society. They are at high risk of educational failure, unemployment, homelessness, imprisonment, and problems in forming stable and satisfactory relationships. They are over-represented in psychiatric care. As a consequence, social policy encourages adoption, fostering and the avoidance of removing children from their parents unless it is necessary for their safety. Children in institutional care usually grow up in reasonable material comfort, but they are impoverished in a more profound way. They have no back-up. Most young adults have little cash to call their own, but in times of hardship can call on assistance from family. This is very different to being absolutely self-reliant. The lives of children who grow up in institutional care are emotionally impoverished by a lack of consistent and loving adults, and this frequently leads to a profound emotional insecurity. They lack a network of reliable support founded on personal affection. They often lack early role models to guide patterns of adult behaviour later in life.

- In Alan's case, insecurity made him solitary. Like many people with similar backgrounds, military service suited him, because it offered security without making emotional demands. It offered clear rules and an unambiguous role. He thrived, and he was then able to form a stable loving relationship, though it was one that cast him into a position of dependency that he saw no need to escape from.

- His relationship with his employers was similarly dependent and static. His emotional needs were now being met by his wife and his job in a way that they had never been met during his childhood, but it was difficult for him to look ahead and recognise that either or both were likely to eventually prove unreliable, and that his adult experience would leave him no better equipped to manage his life on his own than he had been when he joined the Army in his mid teens.

- His experience of illness (his own tuberculosis and his wife's cancer), together with a lack of psychological sophistication borne of an emotionally barren childhood, made it highly likely that when he felt 'wrong' he would experience this as bodily illness, in other words that he would somatise distress. This put him in a state of conflict with his GP, and delayed him getting appropriate help for what eventually became a self-sustaining and life-threatening depressive illness. One might speculate that he had inherited a vulnerability to obsessionality and depression, but there is no need to invoke this in order to make sense of the situation.

- Although he regarded his adult life as entirely satisfactory, it had not helped him to develop a repertoire of behaviours in order to cope with novel and adverse situations. Indeed, his early financial insecurity meant that he could not cope with an unexpected drop in income. When it happened he was paralysed by worry and he could not deploy his income effectively.

- All of these factors can be seen to have come together to make him feel that his situation was hopeless, and that suicide was the only way of resolving his problems.

Narrative is not the only way to bring the biological, psychological and social together, but it is a familiar and clinically useful way of understanding life. It provides a link between science, clinical practice and the problems in individual patients' lives, and as such it is a tool of applied scientific empiricism. Using narrative demands an understanding of history-taking as a dynamic and continuing task. If history is understood as a handful of facts under a series of headings on an assessment proforma, then it is unlikely to be meaningful. History needs to be returned to, re-evaluated and understood as treatment proceeds, so that it becomes a coherent narrative, jointly owned by patient and clinician.

Main points in this chapter

1. Working with poverty demands that the clinician is mindful of power imbalances and class differences that can sabotage therapeutic relationships.
2. Clinicians have to be open to learning about the lifestyle and culture of people who may be living very different lives to themselves.
3. Deprived people may not automatically trust authority figures. Treatment is more likely to be successful if trust is earned through openness, honesty and a disinclination to patronise.
4. Psychiatry has to follow a balanced biopsychosocial approach because, whilst biological, psychological and social perspectives each contribute to science and clinical practice, none of them offers the possibility of a comprehensive way of understanding and relieving mental illness.
5. Social psychiatry has a number of distinctive characteristics. These are set out.
6. Narrative is an important way of bringing together the diverse factors that cause and shape mental illness. It has usefulness in planning treatment for individual patients. It is also a tool for scientific understanding.

Afterword

Finally, we are going to speculate a little and explore some public health and social policy implications of the relationship between mental health and poverty.

In various places we have been critical of a range of ideas about mental illness and its management. In some cases, we accept the validity of the ideas, but we do not believe they offer an overarching solution to mental health problems. In other cases, we have been more strident. There are some threads in contemporary thinking about mental illness that we believe to be seriously flawed. Post-modernism is one example. This tradition has been valuable in providing an awareness of the importance of values and, through the work of Kuhn and others, in drawing attention to the role of paradigms or meta-models. However, some post-modernists are dismissive of any validity in ideas of truth and objectivity. In our opinion, this is against reason and it is a complete dead-end in trying to understand the world.

We hope that we have not seemed overly negative, as an intention behind this book is to draw out evidence that change is possible for society and individuals. Our understanding of the current state of knowledge about mental health leads us to believe that there are good grounds for optimism, albeit tempered by the awareness that there are political obstacles to be overcome. We believe the incidence and prevalence of mental illness can be reduced in the foreseeable future. To achieve this, there is a need to create a hopeful consensus about preventative public health measures in the form of social change that can be implemented in the here and now. Consensus cannot be built upon the hegemony of a single set of ideas. It demands general agreement across the spectrum of scientific orientation that certain measures would be highly likely to work.

We have defended some unpopular concepts, such as the medical model. Two of us are doctors and our background in medicine influences our thinking. The medical model is so reviled that it is easy to overlook the importance of understanding biomedical aspects of mental illness, including the interaction of physical and mental health. Attacks on the medical model tend to be based on a crude characterisation of doctors as obsessed with biology and as being in the pocket of the pharmaceutical industry. This may be true of some psychiatrists, but it is not generally true. It is not scientifically valid to dismiss all medical approaches by reference to practitioners corrupted by Pharma or doctors who hold unusual and untenable beliefs. There is a medical model that we believe is entirely defensible (Poole & Higgo, 2006), reflected in the fact that psychotherapy, public health, social therapy and therapeutic communities all had their origins in medicine and remain part of its intellectual traditions.

We do not suggest that any version of the medical model should take precedence over other ways of understanding mental disorders. On the contrary, a struggle to reduce inequality in the interests of mental health should be led by people diagnosed with mental illness themselves, supported by the mental health professions. Unfortunately, the mental health professions are sometimes self-indulgently schismatic. For example, there is a faction within clinical psychology that continues to set up psychiatry as an Aunt Sally and attack it. It includes some empirical scientists, such as Richard Bentall, who has written a book called *Doctoring the Mind: Why Psychiatric Treatments Fail* (Bentall, 2009). At the time of writing, the British Psychological Society Clinical Psychology Division have recently issued a position paper (British Psychological Society, 2013) that rejects 'the disease model' and 'functional psychiatric diagnoses' in their entirety, calling for a 'paradigm shift' to psychological formulation. This would be, the document claims, more evidence-based and humane.

These skirmishes seem to us to have everything to do with professional tensions, and nothing to do with meeting the needs of people with mental health problems. One-to-one psychological approaches are the core strength of clinical psychology, and they are very powerful under some circumstances. However, one-to-one talking treatments do not offer a solution to everything. Nothing does. The provision of effective services for people with complex problems that arise out of adversity and disadvantage requires team work from professionals from a number of different disciplines. A broad campaign to reduce inequality will be sabotaged if there are battles in the background over which profession has the best model. There is no best model.

We have seen that poverty is bad for mental health across the board. Poverty is, however, a complex phenomenon that involves more than just a lack of cash. Not all poverty is equal, and childhood exposure to inner-city poverty is particularly bad for mental health. The magnitude of the specific effect of an inner-city childhood varies between disorders. For one particular indicator of mental health, there is a reversal of this general trend; suicide is commoner in the countryside. In the case of schizophrenia, there is a consensus that social factors have an aetiological role (e.g. Boydell *et al.*, 2004b). Social environment has come to be seen as a major cause of mental illness. This is a mainstream belief amongst schizophrenia researchers. There is the possibility of general agreement that a key element in the prevention of schizophrenia might be action to reduce the number of children growing up in poverty, and especially in urban poverty. Wilkinson and Pickett (2009) have argued that a wide range of social and health problems have an intimate relationship with income inequality. They suggest that addressing inequality is the key intervention to reduce rates of a broad range of health and social problems in the UK.

Despite some tantalising and suggestive findings, and a number of theories, it is far from clear what specific elements of living in poverty and inner cities are damaging. The explanations that can be offered are largely speculative. More important than the precise mechanisms is the question of whether it is possible to do anything about the mental health consequences of poverty. On the one hand, this would inevitably mean reducing social inequality in general. On the other hand, it might involve intervention to eliminate severe inner-city poverty as a particular feature of large cities. One can object that we do not know for sure that such changes would be effective. Set against this, many other medical and social problems are likely to be positively affected, and sometimes you just have to try something new.

There are precedents here. Effective public health interventions have been implemented in the absence of knowledge of explanatory mechanisms. For example, in 1854, John Snow did not need to have a bacteriological understanding of cholera in order to conclude that an outbreak in London was being transmitted through the water supply. It was sufficient to use local information and statistics to conclude that there was a correlation between clinical cases of cholera and the consumption of water supplied by a particular company. As it happens, preventing access to that water probably was not critical in ending the epidemic of cholera. The number of new cases was already in decline when he removed the handle from the Broad Street pump. However, his work on the epidemic established the foundations of epidemiology in public health. It was long after this, in 1885, that Robert Koch identified *Vibrio Cholerae* as the pathogenic micro-organism. What Snow recognised was the likely existence of a responsible pathogenic agent in the water supply.

One of the main objections to the reduction or elimination of poverty is that it is a utopian objective that is unattainable. There is a body of opinion that regards the existence of a very deprived group in society as inevitable. Jesus Christ is reported to have said 'For ye have the poor always with you' (Matthew 26:11), which is often taken to support the inevitability of some people being poor. The modern argument runs to the effect that all societies are bound to have a group at the bottom, who are equally bound to experience a disproportionate burden of social and health problems. However, international comparisons demonstrate that there are major differences in the extent of income inequality, which suggests that mitigation of the effects of poverty is possible, even if complete elimination of it is not.

There is a further objection to the egalitarian position, where it is argued that the existence of a relatively small impoverished population is a price worth paying in order to reap the rewards of the massive productive power of unrestricted market capitalism. However, it is not necessary to completely overthrow capitalism, as it can function without maximal profitability. Wilkinson and Pickett point out that greater equality is achieved within capitalism in the Scandinavian countries, amongst other international and historical examples. They argue that the whole population suffers ill effects from wide inequality and that the benefits of unrestricted profit making are illusory.

If there is one thing that we should learn from the Recovery movement, it is the importance of hope. At the time of writing we are five years into an unprecedented global depression, the effects of which are projected to continue for at least as long again, if not forever. The political rhetoric states that the only way forward is austerity in public services, meaning the removal of protection for the most vulnerable people in British society, and a maximisation of profitability for big business, in the expectation that this will lead to the return of unrestrained economic growth. For millions of people this is a message of despair. They are going to become poorer, not wealthier, and there is no other way forward. We need more hope than this in our lives, both individually and collectively.

Fortunately, the *despair-is-the-only-way-forward* argument is nonsense. There are alternative strategies. There are costs to one section of society or another, no matter what economic policy is followed. There is no intrinsic reason why the burden of the present crisis should disproportionately fall on the poor. The evidence strongly suggests that maximising growth and profitability is not the optimal strategy for whole populations. It is particularly odd to argue that there is no way forward other than unrestricted neo-liberal policies when it is clear that it was the pursuit of such policies that caused the economic crisis in the first place.

Austerity and growing inequality cannot be accepted as inevitable and somehow necessary for the public good. As physicians and scientists we have access to clear evidence that there are other ways forward. We know that less profitability could mean greater well-being. We know that decreasing income inequality and improving the quality of inner-city life could reduce the unacceptably high rates of severe mental illness in some sections of the population. We know that these are not utopian objectives but attainable goals. Far from straying into the political arena, bringing these facts to attention is simply a matter of speaking truth to power.

Above all, hope springs from control over one's own destiny. At an individual level this is an important component of Recovery. Grasping some control is a necessary step to allow people in poverty collectively to improve their lot. People diagnosed with mental illness need to take the lead in demanding better, more appropriate services, and people living in poverty need to take the lead in demanding change in social and economic policies. The role of clinicians and scientists is to support them by providing the evidence, even where this involves telling policy makers things that they don't want to hear.

References

Allardyce J, Boydell J, Van Os J, *et al.* (2001) Comparison of the incidence of schizophrenia in rural Dumfries and Galloway and urban Camberwell. *British Journal of Psychiatry* 179: 335–339.

Allebeck P, Andreasson S (1996) Drug induced psychosis. *British Journal of Psychiatry* 169: 114–115.

Altamura AC, Goodwin GM (2010) How Law 180 in Italy has reshaped psychiatry after 30 years: past attitudes, current trends and unmet needs. *British Journal of Psychiatry* 197: 261–262.

Amodio DM (2010) Can neuroscience advance social psychological theory? Social neuroscience for the behavioural social psychologist. *Social Cognition* 28: 695–716.

Andreasson S, Allebeck P, Engstrom A, Rydberg U (1987) Cannabis and schizophrenia. A longitudinal study of Swedish conscripts. *Lancet* 330: 1483–1486.

Anthony WA (1993) Recovery from mental illness: the guiding vision of the mental health service system in the 1990s. *Psychosocial Rehabilitation Journal* 16: 11–23.

Arendt M, Rosenberg R, Foldager L, Perto G, Munk-Jørgensen P (2005) Cannabis induced psychosis and subsequent schizophrenia-spectrum disorders: follow-up of 535 incident cases. *British Journal of Psychiatry* 18: 510–515.

Arseneault L, Cannon M, Poulton R, *et al.* (2002) Cannabis use in adolescence and risk for adult psychosis: longitudinal prospective study. *British Medical Journal* 325: 1212–1213.

Babor T, Caetano R, Casswell S, *et al.* (2010) *Alcohol: No Ordinary Commodity*, 2nd edition. Oxford: Oxford University Press.

Bailey J, Poole R, Zinovieff F, *et al.* (2011) *Achieving Positive Change in the Drinking Culture of Wales* Cardiff: Alcohol Concern Cymru.

Barnes T, Hutton SB, Watt H, Joyce E (2006) Co-morbid substance use and age at onset of schizophrenia. *British Journal of Psychiatry* 188: 237–242.

Barrio G, Montanari L, Bravo MJ, *et al.* (2013) Trends of heroin use and heroin injection epidemics in Europe: findings from the EMCDDA treatment demand indicator (TDI). *Journal of Substance Misuse* 45: 19–30.

Barth J, Bermetz L, Heim E, Trelle S, Tonia T (2012) The current prevalence of child sexual abuse worldwide: a systematic review and meta-analysis. *International Journal of Public Health* 58: 469–483.

Bauld L (2011) *The Impact of Smoke-free Legislation in England: Evidence Review*. Bath: University of Bath.

Bentall R (1992) A proposal to classify happiness as a psychiatric disorder. *Journal of Medical Ethics* 18: 94–98.

Bentall R (2004) *Madness Explained: Psychosis and Human Nature*. London: Penguin.

Bentall R (2009) *Doctoring The Mind: Why Psychiatric Treatments Fail*. London: Allen Lane.

Bentall RP, Wickham S, Shevlin M, Varese F (2012) Do specific early-life adversities lead to specific symptoms of psychosis? A study from the 2007 Adult Psychiatric Morbidity Study. *Schizophrenia Bulletin* 38: 734–740.

Beresford P (2010) Re-examining relationships between experience, knowledge, ideas and research: the key role for recipients of state welfare and their movements. *Social Work and Society* 8: 6–21.

Bevan A (1952) *In Place of Fear*. New York: Simon and Schuster, p. 4.

Bhugra D, Leff JP, eds. (1993) *The Principles of Social Psychiatry*. Oxford: Blackwell.

Björkqvist K (2001) Social defeat as a stressor in humans. *Physiology and Behaviour* 73: 435–442.

Black D, Townsend P, Whitehead M, Davidson N (1993) *Inequalities in Health*. London: Penguin Books.

Blakely TA, Collings SCD, Atkinson J (2003) Unemployment and suicide. Evidence for a causal association? *Journal of Epidemiology and Community Health* 57: 594–600.

Booth A, Meier P, Stockwell T, Sutton A, Wilkinson A, Wong R, Taylor K (2008) *Independent Review of the Effects of Alcohol Pricing and Promotion. Part A: Systematic Reviews*. Sheffield: School of Health and Related Research, University of Sheffield.

Bos AER, Pryor JB, Reeder GD, Stutterheim SE (2013) Stigma: advances in theory and research. *Basic and Applied Social Psychology* 35: 1–9.

Bostock Y (2003) *Searching for the Solution: Women, Smoking and Inequalities in Europe*. London: Health Development Agency.

Bourdieu P (1986) The forms of capital, in Richardson, John G, ed., *Handbook of Theory and Research for the Sociology of Education*. New York: Greenwood.

Boydell J, van Os J, McKenzie K, Murray RM (2004a) The association of inequality with the incidence of schizophrenia: an ecological study. *Social Psychiatry and Psychiatric Epidemiology* 39: 597–599.

Boydell J, Van Os J, Murray R (2004b) Is there a role for social factors in a comprehensive developmental model for schizophrenia?, in Keshavan MS, Kennedy JL, Murray RM eds, *Neurodevelopment and Schizophrenia*. Cambridge: Cambridge University Press.

Bracken P, Thomas P (2005) *Post-Psychiatry: Mental Health in a Post-Modern World*. Oxford: Oxford University Press.

Bracken P, Thomas P (2009) Beyond consultation: the challenge of working with user/survivor and carer groups. *Psychiatric Bulletin* 33: 241–243.

Brennan A, Purshous R, Rafia R, Taylor K, Meier P (2008) *Independent Review of the Effects of Alcohol Pricing and Promotion. Part B: Modelling the Potential Impact of Pricing and Promotion Policies for Alcohol in England: Results from the Sheffield Alcohol Policy Model*. Sheffield: School of Health and Related Research, University of Sheffield.

Briere J, Elliott DM (2003) Prevalence and psychological sequelae of self-reported childhood physical and sexual abuse in a general population sample of men and women. *Child Abuse & Neglect* 27: 1205–1222.

British Psychological Society (2013) *Position Statement of Division of Clinical Psychology on the Classification of Behaviour and Experience in Relation to Functional Psychiatric Diagnoses. Time for a Paradigm Shift*. London: British Psychological Society.

Brown G, Harris T (1978) *The Social Origins of Depression: A Study of Psychiatric Disorder in Women*. London: Tavistock.

Burns JK, Esterhuizen T (2008) Poverty, inequality and the treated incidence of first-episode psychosis: an ecological study from South Africa. *Social Psychiatry and Psychiatric Epidemiology* 43: 331–335.

Burns T, Rugkåsa J, Molodynski A, *et al.* (2013) Community treatment orders for patients with psychosis (OCTET): a randomised controlled trial. *The Lancet* 381: 1627–1633.

Burns T, Yeeles K, Molodynski A, *et al.* (2011) Pressures to adhere to treatment ('leverage') in English mental healthcare. *British Journal of Psychiatry* 199: 145–150.

Caspi A, Moffitt T, Cannon M, *et al.* (2005) Moderation of the effect of adolescent-onset cannabis use on adult psychosis by a functional polymorphism in the Catechol-O-Methyltransferase gene: longditudinal evidence of a gene x environment interaction. *Biological Psychiatry* 57: 1117–1127.

Chaux E, Molano A, Podlesky P (2009) Socio-economic, socio-political and socio-emotional variables explaining school bullying: a country-wide multilevel analysis. *Aggressive Behaviour* 35: 520–529.

Clark D (1996) *The Story of a Mental Hospital: Fulbourn 1858–1983*. London: Process Press.

Clark DM, Layard R, Smithies R (2008) Improving access to psychological therapy: initial evaluation of the two demonstration sites. *CEP Discussion Paper 897 Centre for Economic Performance*. London: LSE.

Clarke MC, Harley M, Cannon M (2006) The role of obstetric events in schizophrenia. *Schizophrenia Bulletin* 32: 3–8.

Cohen SI (1996) Substance-induced psychosis. *British Journal of Psychiatry*, 168: 651–652.

Cohen SI, Johnson K (1988) Psychosis from alcohol or drug abuse. *British Medical Journal* 297: 1270–1271.

Coleman LJ, Cross TL (2005) *Being Gifted at School: An Introduction to Development, Guidance and Teaching*. Waco, TX: Pruffrock Press.

Compton WM, Volkow ND (2006) Major increases in opioid analgesic abuse in the United States: concerns and strategies. *Drug and Alcohol Dependence* 81: 103–107.

Connell PH (1958) *Amphetamine Psychosis (Maudsley Monograph Number 5)* Oxford: Oxford University Press.

Cook CCH (2009) Substance misuse, in Cook C, Powell A, Sims A, eds, *Spirituality and Psychiatry*. London: Royal College of Psychiatrists.

Cook CCH, Poole R, Higgo R (2012) Holistic psychiatry. *The Psychiatrist* 36: 235–236.

Corrigan PW, Watson AC (2002) The paradox of self-stigma and mental illness. *Clinical Psychology, Science and Practice* 9: 35–53.

Coulter A (2005) The NHS revolution: health care in the market place. What do patients and the public want from primary care? *British Medical Journal* 331: 1199–1201.

Crabtree JW, Haslam SA, Postmes T, Haslam C (2010) Mental health support groups, stigma and self-esteem: positive and negative implications of group identification. *Journal of Social Issues* 66: 553–569.

Craddock N, Antebi D, Attenburrow M-J, *et al.* (2008) Wake-up call for British psychiatry. *British Journal of Psychiatry* 193: 6–9.

Craddock NJ, Owen MJ (2007) Rethinking psychosis: the disadvantages of a dichotomous classification now outweigh the advantages. *World Psychiatry* 6: 20–27.

Crisp A, Gelder M, Goddard E, Meltzer H (2005) Stigmatisation of people with mental illnesses: a follow-up study within the Changing Minds campaign of the Royal College of Psychiatrists. *World Psychiatry* 4: 106–113.

Cross-Disorder Group of the Psychiatric Genetics Consortium (2013) Identification of risk loci with shared effects on five major psychiatric disorders: a genome-wide analysis. *Lancet* 381: 1371–1379.

Crossley N (1998) RD Laing and the British anti-psychiatry movement: a socio-historical analysis. *Social Science and Medicine* 47: 877–889.

Croudace TJ, Kayne R, Jones PB, Harrison G (2000) Non-linear relationship between an index of social deprivation, psychiatric admission prevalence and the incidence of psychosis. *Psychological Medicine* 30: 177–185.

Crow T (2008) Craddock and Owen vs Kraepelin: 85 years late, mesmerised by "polygenes". *Schizophrenia Research* 103: 156–160.

Culliford L (2011) *The Psychology of Spirituality: An Introduction.* London: Jessica Kingsley.

Curran C, Byrappa N, McBride A (2004) Stimulant psychosis: systematic review. *British Journal of Psychiatry* 185: 196–204.

Davidson K, Roth M (1996) Substance-induced psychosis *British Journal of Psychiatry* 168: 651.

Davidson L, Mezzina R, Rowe M, Thompson K (2010) "A life in the community": Italian mental health reform and recovery. *Journal of Mental Health* 19: 436–43.

Davidson L, O'Connell M, Tondora J, Styron T, Kangas K (2006) The Top Ten concerns about recovery encountered in mental health system transformation. *Psychiatric Services* 57: 640–645.

Dawkins R (1976) *The Selfish Gene.* Oxford: Oxford University Press.

Dawnay E, Shah H (2005) *Behavioural Economics: Seven Principles for Policy-Makers.* London: New Economics Foundation.

Deacon L, Morleo M, Hannon KL, *et al.* (2010) *Alcohol Consumption: Segmentation Series Report 2.* Liverpool: North West Public Health Observatory.

Deegan P (1988) Recovery: the lived experience of rehabilitation. *Psychosocial Rehabilitation Journal* 11: 11–19.

Demyttenaere K, Bruffaerts R, Posada-Villa J, *et al.*; WHO World Mental Health Survey Consortium (2004) Prevalence, severity, and unmet need for treatment of mental disorders in the World Health Organization Mental Health Surveys. *Journal of the American Medical Association* 291: 2581–90.

Department of Health (2001) *The Journey to Recovery: The Government's Vision for Mental Health Care.* London: Department of Health Publications.

Derks B, Inzlicht M, Kang S (2008) The neuroscience of stigma and stereotype threat. *Group Process and Intergroup Relations* 11: 163–181.

Dickens G, Weleminsky J, Onifade Y, Sugarman P (2012) Recovery Star: validating user recovery. *The Psychiatrist* 36: 45–50.

Doll R, Peto R, Wheatley K, Gray R, Sutherland I (1994) Mortality in relation to smoking: 40 years' observations on male British doctors. *British Medical Journal* 309: 901–911.

Edwards G, Gross MM (1976) Alcohol dependence: provisional description of a clinical syndrome. *British Medical Journal* 1 (6017): 1058–1061.

Erskine S, Maheswaran R, Pearson T, and Gleeson D (2010) Socioeconomic deprivation, urban–rural location and alcohol-related mortality in England and Wales. *BMC Public Health* 10: 99.

Evans-Lacko S, Thornicroft G (2010) Stigma among people with dual diagnosis and implications for health services. *Advances in Dual Diagnosis* 3: 4–7.

Faris REL, Dunham HW (1939) *Mental Disorders in Urban Areas.* Chicago: University of Chicago Press.

Fergusson DM, Poulton R, Smith PF, Bowden J (2006) Cannabis and psychosis. *British Medical Journal* 332: 172–175.

Fish FJ (1967) *Clinical Psychopathology: Signs and Symptoms in Psychiatry* (First Edition). Bristol: J Wright.

Fisher HL, Bunn A, Jacobs C, Moran P, Bifulco A (2011a) Concordance between mother and offspring retrospective reports of childhood adversity. *Childhood Abuse and Neglect* 35: 117–122.

Fisher HL, Craig TK, Fearon P, *et al.* (2011b) Reliability and comparability of psychosis patients retrospective reports of childhood abuse. *Schizophrenia Bulletin* 37: 546–553.

Flegr J, Preiss M, Klose J, *et al.* (2003) Decreased level of psychobiological factor novelty seeking and lower intelligence in men latently infected with the protozoan parasite *Toxaplasma Gondii*: dopamine a missing link between schizophrenia and toxoplasmosis. *Biological Psychology* 63: 253–268.

Fone DL, Dunstan F, John A, Lloyd K (2007) Associations between common mental disorders and the Mental Illness Needs Index in community settings. *British Journal of Psychiatry* 191: 158–163.

Ford T, Vostanis P, Meltzer H, Goodman R (2007) Psychiatric disorder among British children looked after by local authorities: comparison with children living in private households. *British Journal of Psychiatry* 190: 319–325.

Foucault M (2005) *Madness and Civilisation: A History of Insanity in the Age of Reason.* Oxford: Routledge.

French RV (1884) *Nineteen Centuries of Drink in England: A History.* London: National Temperance Publication Depot.

Ghaemi SN (2009) The rise and fall of the biopsychosocial model. *British Journal of Psychiatry* 195: 3–4.

Glover GR, Leese M, McCrone P (1999) More severe mental illness is more concentrated in deprived areas. *British Journal of Psychiatry* 175: 544–548.

Glover GR, Robin E, Emami J, Arabscheibani GR (1998) A needs index for mental health care. *Social Psychiatry and Psychiatric Epidemiology* 33: 89–96.

Goffman E (1961) *Asylums: Essays on the Social Situation of Mental Patients and Other Inmates.* New York: Anchor.

Goffman E (1963) *Stigma: Notes on the Management of Spoiled Identity.* New York: Simon & Schuster.

Goldberg EM, Morrison SL (1963) Schizophrenia and social class. *British Journal of Psychiatry* 109: 785–802.

Goodman LA, Rosenberg SD, Mueser KT, Drake RE (1997) Physical and sexual assault history in women with serious mental illness: prevalence, correlates, treatment and future directions. *Schizophrenia Bulletin* 23: 685–696.

Graham H (2012) Smoking, stigma and social class. *Journal of Social Policy* 41: 83–99.

Grinshpoon A, Barchana M, Ponizovsky A, *et al.* (2005) Cancer in schizophrenia: is the risk higher or lower? *Schizophrenia Research* 73: 333–341.

Haines VA, Beggs JJ, Hulbert JS (2011) Neighbourhood disadvantage, network social capital and depressive symptoms. *Journal of Health and Social Behaviour* 52: 58–73.

Hamilton M (ed.) (1984) *Fish's Schizophrenia*, 3rd edition. Bristol: PSG Wright.

Hammersley P, Dias A, Tood G, *et al.* (2003) Childhood trauma and hallucinations in bipolar affective disorder: preliminary investigation. *British Journal of Psychiatry* 182: 543–547.

Harding J, Irving A, Whowell M (2011) *Homelessness, Pathways to Exclusion and Opportunities for Intervention.* Newcastle-upon-Tyne: Northumbria Graphics, Arts and Social Sciences Academic Press.

Hare EH (1956) Mental illness and social conditions in Bristol. *Journal of Mental Science* 102: 349–357.

Harris M, Farquhar F, Healy D, *et al.* (2011) The incidence and prevalence of admissions for melancholia in two cohorts (1875–1924 and 1995–2005). *Journal of Affective Disorders* 134: 45–51.

Harrison G, Amin S, Singh SP, Croudace T, Jones P (1999) Outcome of psychosis in people of African–Caribbean family origin. *British Journal of Psychiatry* 175: 43–49.

Harrison G, Gunnell D, Glazebrook C, Page K, Kwiecinski R (2001a) Association between schizophrenia and social inequality at birth: case–control study. *British Journal of Psychiatry* 179: 346–350.

Harrison G, Hopper K, Craig T, *et al.* (2001b) Recovery from psychotic illness: a 15- and 25-year international follow-up study. *British Journal of Psychiatry* 178: 506–517.

Hasson-Ohayon I, Levy I, Kravetz S, Vollanski-Narkis A, Roe D (2011) Insight into mental illness, self-stigma, and the family burden of person with a severe mental illness. *Comprehensive Psychiatry* 52: 75–80.

Hastings G, Brooks O, Stead M, Angus K, Anker T, Farrell T (2010) Alcohol advertising: the last chance saloon. *British Medical Journal* 340: 184–186.

Health and Social Care Information Centre (2012) *Prescriptions Dispensed in the Community: England, Statistics for 2001 to 2011.* London: NHS HSCIC.

Health and Social Care Information Centre, Community and Mental Health Team (2012) *Inpatients Formally Detained in Hospitals Under the Mental Health Act 1983, and Patients Subject to Supervised Community Treatment, Annual Figures, England, 2011/12.* London: Health and Social Care Information Centre.

Herron J, Cehurstm H, Appleby L, Perry A, Cordingley L (2001) Attitudes toward suicide prevention in front-line health staff. *Suicide and Life-Threatening Behavior* 31: 342–347.

Hills J (2010) *An Anatomy of Economic Inequality in the UK: Report of the National Equality Panel.* London: London School of Economics.

Hopper K (2007) Rethinking social recovery in schizophrenia: what a capabilities approach might offer. *Society, Science and Medicine* 65: 868–879.

Hopper K, Harrison G, Janca A, Sartorius N (eds) (2007) *Recovery from Schizophrenia: An International Perspective. A Report from the WHO Collaborative Project, The International Study of Schizophrenia.* Oxford: Oxford University Press.

Hossenbaccus Z, White PD (2013) Views on the nature of chronic fatigue syndrome: content analysis. *Journal of Royal Society of Medicine Short Reports* 4: 1–6.

Houghton, J (1982) Maintaining mental health in a turbulent world. *Schizophrenia Bulletin* 8: 548–552.

Hutchinson G, Takei N, Fahy TA, *et al.* (1996) Morbid risk of schizophrenia in first degree relatives of White and African–Caribbean patients with psychosis. *British Journal of Psychiatry* 169: 776–780.

International Schizophrenia Consortium, Purcell SM, Wray NR, Stone JL, *et al.* (2009) Common polygenic variation contributes to risk of schizophrenia and bipolar disorder. *Nature* 460: 748–52.

Isbell H, Gorodetzsky CW, Jasinski D, Claussen U, von Spulak F, Korte F (1967) Effects of Delta 9-transtetrahydrocannabinol in man. *Psychopharmacologia* 11: 691–696.

Jarman B (1984) Underprivileged areas: validation and distribution of scores. *British Medical Journal* 289: 1587–1592.

Jauhar S, Smith ID (2009) Alcohol related brain damage: not a silent epidemic. *British Journal of Psychiatry* 194: 287–288.

Jefferis BJ, Manor O, Power C (2007) Social gradients in binge drinking and abstaining: trends in a cohort of British adults. *Journal of Epidemiology and Community Health* 61: 150–153.

Jones O (2012) *Chavs: the Demonization of the Working Class.* London: Verso.

Käsler D (1989) *Max Weber: An Introduction to His Life and Work.* Chicago: University of Chicago Press.

Kelly BD, O'Callaghan E, Waddington JL, *et al.* (2010) Schizophrenia and the city: a review of literature and prospective study of psychosis and urbanicity in Ireland. *Schizophrenia Research* 116: 75–89.

Kendell RE (1976) The classification of depressions: a review of contemporary confusion. *British Journal of Psychiatry* 129: 15–28.

Killaspy H, Meier R (2010) A Fair Deal for mental health includes local rehabilitation services. *The Psychiatrist* 34: 265–267.

Kinney DK, Teixeira P, Hsu D, *et al.* (2009) Relation of schizophrenia prevalence to latitude, climate, fish consumption, infant mortality and skin colour: a role for prenatal vitamin D deficiency and infections? *Schizophrenia Bulletin* 35: 582–595.

Kirkbride JB, Errazuriz A, Croudace TJ, *et al.* (2012a) Incidence of schizophrenia and other psychoses in England, 1950–2009: a systematic review and meta-analyses. *PLoS ONE* 7(3): e31660. doi:10.1371/journal.pone.0031660.

Kirkbride JB, Morgan C, Fearon P, *et al.* (2007) Neighbourhood-level effects on psychoses: re-examining the role of context. *Psychological Medicine* 37: 1413–25.

Kirkbride JB, Stubbins C, Jones PB (2012b) Psychosis incidence through the prism of early intervention services. *British Journal of Psychiatry* 200: 156–157.

Komuravelli A, Poole R, Higgo R (2011) Stability of the diagnosis of first-episode drug-induced psychosis. *The Psychiatrist* 35: 224–227.

Krabbendam L, Van Os J (2005) Schizophrenia and urbanicity: a major environmental influence – conditional on genetic risk. *Schizophrenia Bulletin* 31: 795–799.

Krayer A, Robinson CA, Poole R, Wolfendale C, Zinovieff F (2013) *Service Provision for People with Mental Health and Substance Misuse Problems – the Relationship Between Stigma and Social Exclusion.* Final report to National Institute for Social Care and Health Research, Bangor University.

Kuhn T (1996) *The Structure of Scientific Revolutions*, 3rd edition. Chicago: University of Chicago Press.

Kusow A, Wilson LC, Martin DE (1997) Determinants of citizen satisfaction with police: the effects of residential location. *Policing: An International Journal of Police Strategy and Management* 20: 655–664.

Laing RD (1965) *The Divided Self: An Existential Study in Sanity and Madness.* London: Penguin.

Laing RD (1967) *The Politics of Experience and the Bird of Paradise.* London: Penguin.

Lasser K, Boyd W, Woolhandler S, Himmelstein DU, McCormick D, Bor DH (2000) Smoking and mental illness: a population based prevalence study. *Journal of the American Medical Association* 248: 2606–2610.

Laugharne R, Priebe S (2006) Trust, choice and power in mental health: a literature review. *Social Psychiatry and Psychiatric Epidemiology* 41: 843–852.

Layard R (1980) Human satisfactions and public policy. *The Economic Journal* 90: 737–770.

Layard R, Clark D, Knapp M, Mayraz G (2007) Cost–benefit analysis of psychological therapy. *Journal of the National Institute of Economic and Social Research* 202: 90–98.

Leete E (1988) The treatment of schizophrenia: a patient's perspective. *Hospital and Community Psychiatry* 38: 486–491.

Leon D, McCambridge J (2006) Liver cirrhosis mortality rates in Britain from 1950 to 2002: an analysis of routine data. *Lancet* 367: 52–56.

Lepping P, Malik M (2013) Community treatment orders: current practice and a framework to aid clinicians. *The Psychiatrist* 37: 54–57.

Levin KA, Leyland AH (2005) Urban/rural inequalities in suicide in Scotland, 1981–1999. *Social Science and Medicine* 60: 2877–2890.

Lewis AJ (1934) Melancholia: a clinical survey of depressive states. *Journal of Mental Science* 80: 277–378.

Lewis G, David A, Andréasson S, Allebeck P (1992) Schizophrenia and city life. *Lancet* 340: 137–140.

Lewontin RC, Rose S, Kamin LJ (1984) *Not In Our Genes: Biology, Ideology and Human Nature.* New York: Pantheon Books.

Lichlyter B, Purdon S, Tibbo P (2011) Predictors of psychosis severity in individuals with primary stimulant addictions. *Addictive Behaviours* 36: 137–139.

Lichtenstein P, Yip BH, Bjork C, *et al.* (2009) Common genetic determinants of schizophrenia and bipolar disorder in Swedish families: a population based study. *Lancet* 373: 234–9.

Lifton RJ (1986) *The Nazi Doctors: Medical Killing and the Psychology of Genocide.* New York: Basic Books.

Linden SC, Jackson MC, Subramanian L, Healy D, Linden D (2011) Sad benefit in face working memory: an emotional bias of melancholic depression. *Journal of Affective Disorders* 135: 251–257.

Link BJ, Phelan JC, Bresnahan M, Stueve A, Pescosolido BA (1999) Public conceptions of mental illness: labels, causes, dangerousness and social distance. *American Journal of Public Health* 89: 1328–1333.

Lowry RJ, Billett A, Buchanan C, Whiston S (2009) Increasing breast feeding and reducing smoking in pregnancy: a social marketing success improving life chances for children. *Perspectives in Public Health* 129: 277–280.

Luhrmann TM (2007) Social defeat and the culture of chronicity: or, why schizophrenia does so well over there and so badly here. *Culture, Medicine and Psychiatry* 31: 135–172.

Mackenbach JP (2002) Income inequality and population health. *British Medical Journal* 324: 1–2.

Maj M (2005) 'Psychiatric co-morbidity': an artefact of current diagnostic systems? *British Journal of Psychiatry* 186: 182–184.

Mandelbrote BM (1965) The use of psychodynamic and sociodynamic principles in treatment of psychotics: a change from ward unit concepts to grouped communities. *Comprehensive Psychiatry* 6: 381–387.

Mandelbrote BM, Folkard S (1961) Some factors related to outcome and social adjustment in schizophrenia. *Acta Psychiatrica Scandavica* 37: 223–235.

Mandiberg JM, Warner R (2013) Is mainstreaming always the answer? The social and economic development of service user communities. *The Psychiatrist* 37: 153–155.

Marmot M (1997) Inequality, deprivation and alcohol use. *Addiction* 92 Suppl 1: S13–20.

Marmot M (2005) Social determinants of health inequalities. *Lancet* 365: 1099–1104.

Martin J, Pescosolido BA, Tuch SA (2000) Of fear and loathing: the role of 'disturbing behaviour', labels, and causal attributions in shaping public attitudes of people with mental illness. *Journal of Health and Social Behaviour* 41: 208–223.

Marx K, Engels F (2008) *The Communist Manifesto*. London: Pluto Press.

McConnell KJ, Gast SHN, Ridgely MS, *et al.* (2012) Behavioural health insurance parity: does Oregon's experience presage the national experience with the Mental Health Parity and Addiction Equity Act? *American Journal of Psychiatry* 169: 31–38.

McCulloch A (2012) Housing density as a predictor of neighbourhood satisfaction among families with young children in urban England. *Population, Space and Place* 18: 85–99.

McPherson S, Evans C, Richardson P (2009) The NICE depression guidelines and the recovery model: is there an evidence base for IAPT? *Journal of Mental Health* 18: 405–414.

Melle I (2013) The Breivik case and what psychiatrists can learn from it. *World Psychiatry* 12: 16–21.

Mittal VA, Ellman LM, Cannon TD (2008) Gene–environment interaction and covariation in schizophrenia: the role of obstetric complications. *Schizophrenia Bulletin* 34: 1083–1094.

Moncrieff J (2006) Psychiatric drug promotion and the politics of neoliberalism. *British Journal of Psychiatry* 188: 301–302.

Montoya J, Liesenfeld O (2004) Toxoplasmosis. *Lancet* 363: 1965–1976.

Moore THW, Zammit S, Lingford-Hughes A, *et al.* (2007) Cannabis use and risk of psychotic or affective mental health outcomes: a systematic review. *Lancet* 370: 319–328.

Moorina RE, Holmana CDJ, Garfield C, Bramelda KJ (2006) Health related migration: evidence of reduced "urban-drift". *Health & Place* 12: 131–140.

Morgan C, Curran V (2008) Effects of cannabidiol on schizophrenia-like symptoms in people who use cannabis. *British Journal of Psychiatry* 192: 306–307.

Morgan C, Hutchinson G (2010) The social determinants of psychosis in migrant and ethnic minority populations: a public health tragedy. *Psychological Medicine* 40: 705–709.

Morleo M, Dedman D, O'Farrell I, *et al.* (2010a) *Alcohol-attributable Hospital Admissions: Segmentation Series Report 3*. Liverpool: North West Public Health Observatory.

Morleo M, Spalding J, Carlin H, *et al.* (2010b) *Alcohol Pen Portraits: Segmentation Series Report 4*. Liverpool: North West Public Health Observatory.

Morrice JKW (1966) Dingleton Hospital's therapeutic community. *Psychiatric Services* 17: 140–143.

Mortensen P, Pedersen C, Melbye M, Mors O, Ewald H (2003) Individual and familial risk factors for bipolar affective disorders in Denmark. *Archives of General Psychiatry* 60: 1209–1215.

Moynihan R, Heath I, Henry D (2002) Selling sickness: the pharmaceutical industry and disease mongering. *British Medical Journal* 324: 886–891.

Muller A (2002) Education, income inequality and mortality: a multiple regression analysis. *British Medical Journal* 324: 23–25.

Murphy K, Cherney A (2012) Understanding co-operation with police in a diverse society. *British Journal of Criminology* 52: 181–201.

Murray R, Goldberg D (2006) *The Maudsley Handbook of Practical Psychiatry.* Oxford: Oxford University Press.

National Collaborating Centre for Mental Health (2010) *Depression: The Treatment and Management of Depression in Adults (National Clinical Practice Guideline 90).* London: National Institute for Health and Clinical Excellence.

National Evaluation of Sure Start Team (2010) The impact of Sure Start Local Programmes on five year olds and their families. *Research Report DFE-RR067.* London: Department for Education.

Nicholson LA (2008) Rural mental health. *Advances in Psychiatric Treatment* 14: 302–311.

Nielsen SF, Hjorthøj CR, Erlangsen A, Nordentoft M (2011) Psychiatric disorders and mortality among people in homeless shelters in Denmark: a nationwide register-based cohort study. *Lancet* 377: 2205–2214.

Niemi-Pynttäri JA, Sund R, Putkonen H, *et al.* (2013) Substance-induced psychoses converting into schizophrenia: a register-based study of 18,478 Finnish inpatient cases. *Journal of Clinical Psychiatry* 74 (1): e94-e99.

Nisbett RE, Aronson J, Blair C, *et al.* (2012) Intelligence: new findings and theoretical developments. *American Psychologist* 67: 130–159.

Nutt DJ, King LA, Phillips LD (2010) Drug harms in the UK: a multicriteria decision analysis. *Lancet* 376: 1558–1565.

Office for National Statistics (2006) *Smoking and Drinking Amongst Adults. General Household Survey 2005.* London: ONS.

Office for National Statistics (2008) *Alcohol Related Deaths In the United Kingdom Statistical Bulletin 2008.* London: ONS.

Office for National Statistics (2009) *Adult Psychiatric Morbidity in England 2007: Results of a Household Survey.* London: ONS.

Orwell G (2001) *The Road to Wigan Pier.* London: Penguin Classics.

Osborn DJ, Levy G, Nazareth I, *et al.* (2007) Relative risk of cardiovascular and cancer mortality in people with severe mental illness from the United Kingdom's General Practice Research Database. *Archives of General Psychiatry* 64: 242–249.

Osler M, Prescott E, Gronbaek M, *et al.* (2002) Income inequality, individual income and mortality in Danish adults: analysis of pooled data from two cohort studies. *British Medical Journal* 324: 13–16.

Park A, Curtice J, Thomson K, Bromley C, Phillips M (2005) *British Social Attitudes: The 21st Report.* London: Sage.

Paykel ES (2003) Life events and affective disorders *Acta Psychiatrica Scandinavica* 108: 61–66.

Peck DF (2005) Foot and mouth outbreak: lessons for mental heath services. *Advances in Psychiatric Treatment* 11: 270–276.

Pedersen CB, Mortensen PB (2001) Evidence of a dose response relationship between urbanicity during upbringing and schizophrenia risk. *Archives of General Psychiatry* 58: 1039–46.

Pedersen CB, Raaschou-Nielsen O, Hertel O, Mortensen PB (2004). Air pollution from traffic and schizophrenia risk. *Schizophrenia Research* 66: 83–85.

Peet M, Horrobin DF (2002) A dose-ranging exploratory study of the effects of ethyl-eicosapentaenoate in patients with persistent schizophrenic symptoms. *Journal of Psychiatric Research* 36: 7–18.

Perkins R (2001) What constitutes success? The relative priority of service users' and clinicians' views of mental health services. *British Journal of Psychiatry* 179: 9–10.

Pescosolido B (2013) The public stigma of mental illness: what do we think; what do we know; what can we prove? *Journal of Health and Social Behaviour* 54: 1–21.

Pescosolido BA, Fettes DL, Martin JK, Monahan J, McLeod JD (2007) Perceived dangerousness of children with mental health problems and support for coerced treatment. *Psychiatric Services* 58: 619–625.

Pescosolido BA, Martin JK, Long S, *et al.* (2010) 'A disease like any other'? A decade of change in public reactions to schizophrenia, depression and alcohol dependence. *American Journal of Psychiatry* 167: 1321–1330.

Philo G, Secker J, Platt S, *et al.* (1994) The impact of the mass media on public images of mental illness: media content and audience belief. *Health Education Journal* 53: 271–281.

Pilgrim D (2008) Recovery and current mental health policy. *Chronic Illness* 4: 295–304.

Pitman A, Caine E (2012) The role of the high-risk approach in suicide prevention. *British Journal of Psychiatry* 201: 175–177.

Poole R, Brabbins C (1996) Drug induced psychosis. *British Journal of Psychiatry* 168: 135–138.

Poole R, Cook C (2011) Praying with a patient constitutes a breach of professional boundaries in psychiatric practice. *British Journal of Psychiatry* 199: 94–98.

Poole R, Fleming A (2005) An evaluation of intensive case finding and assertive outreach in order to improve uptake of medical and psychiatric services amongst the homeless with mental health problems. Cheshire and Merseyside Strategic Health Authority.

Poole R, Higgo R (2006) *Psychiatric Interviewing and Assessment.* Cambridge: Cambridge University Press.

Poole R, Higgo R (2008) *Clinical Skills in Psychiatric Treatment.* Cambridge: Cambridge University Press.

Poole R, Higgo R (2009) Postmodernism and psychiatry. *Psychiatric Bulletin* 33: 481–482.

Poole R, Higgo R (2011) Spirituality and the threat to therapeutic boundaries in psychiatric practice. *Mental Health, Religion and Culture* 14: 19–29.

Poole R, Ryan T, Pearsall A (2002) The NHS, the private sector, and the virtual asylum. *British Medical Journal* 325: 349–350.

Prochaska JJ (2011) Smoking and mental illness: breaking the link. *New England Journal of Medicine* 365: 196–198.

Radhakrishnan M, Hammond G, Jones P, *et al.* (2013) Cost of Improving Access to Psychological Therapies (IAPT) programme: an analysis of cost of session, treatment and recovery in selected Primary Care Trusts in the East of England region. *Behaviour Research and Therapy* 51: 37–45.

Read J, Agar K, Argylle N, Aderhold V (2003) Sexual and physical abuse during childhood and adulthood as predictors of hallucinations, delusions and thought disorder. *Psychology and Psychotherapy: Theory Research and Practice* 76: 1–22.

Read J, Argylle N (1999) Hallucinations, delusions and thought disorder among adult psychiatric inpatients with a history of childhood abuse. *Psychiatric Services* 50: 1467–1472.

Read J, Fraser A (1998) Abuse histories of psychiatric inpatients: to ask or not to ask? *Psychiatric Services* 49: 355–359.

Reed H (2009). *The Effects of Increasing Tobacco Taxation: A Cost Benefit and Public Finances Analysis.* London: Action on Smoking and Health.

Richardson K, Crosier A (2001) *Smoking and Health Inequalities.* London: Action on Smoking and Health/Health Development Agency.

Riva M, Bambra C, Curtis S, Gauvin L (2010) Collective resources of local social inequalities? Examining the social determinants of mental health in rural areas. *European Journal of Public Health* 21: 197–203.

Roberts G, Wolfson P (2004) The rediscovery of recovery: open to all. *Advances in Psychiatric Treatment* 10: 37–48.

Rogers A, Pilgrim D (2001) *Mental Health Policy in Britain,* 2nd edition. London: Palgrave.

Romme MA, Escher, AD (1989) Hearing voices. *Schizophrenia Bulletin* 15: 209–216.

Room R (2005) Stigma, social inequality and alcohol and drug use. *Drug and Alcohol Review* 24: 143–155.

Rosen A, Stein LI, McGorry P, *et al.* (2013) Specialist community teams backed by years of quality research. *The Psychiatrist* 37: 38.

Rosenquist JN, Fowler JH, Christakis NA (2011) Social network determinants of depression. *Molecular Psychiatry* 16: 273–281.

Roth P (1996) *Sabbath's Theatre.* London: Vintage.

Roychowdhury A (2011) Bridging the gap between risk and recovery: a human needs approach. *The Psychiatrist* 35: 68–73.

Rusch N, Corrigan PW, Todd AR, Bodenhausen GV (2010) Implicit self-stigma in people with mental illness. *Journal of Nervous and Mental Disease* 198: 150–153.

Ryan T, Davies G, Bennet A, Meier R, Killaspy H (2011) *In Sight and In Mind: A Toolkit to Reduce the Use of Out of Area Mental Health Services.* London: Royal College of Psychiatrists

Ryan T, Hatfield B, Sharma I, Simpson V, McIntyre A (2007) A census study of independent mental health sector usage across seven Strategic Health Authorities. *Journal of Mental Health* 16: 243–253.

Ryan T, Pearsall A, Hatfield B, Poole R (2004) Long term care for serious mental illness outside the NHS: a study of out of area placements. *Journal of Mental Health* 13: 435–429.

Salokangas RKR, Heinimaa M, Svirskis T, *et al.* (2009) Perceived negative attitude of others as an early sign of psychosis. *European Psychiatry* 24: 233–238.

Samele C, van Os J, McKenzie K, *et al.* (2001) Does socio-economic status predict course and outcome in patients with psychosis? *Social Psychiatry and Psychiatric Epidemiology* 36: 373–381.

Savage M, Silva E, Warde A (2010) Dis-identification and class identity, in Silva E, Warde A, eds. *Cultural Analysis and Bourdieu's Legacy.* London: Routledge.

Schneider B, Remillard C (2013) Caring about homelessness: how identity work maintains the stigma of homelessness. *Text and Talk* 33: 95–112.

Scruton R (2000) Bring back stigma. *City Journal* 10: 68–75.

Seddon T (2006) Drugs, crime and social exclusion: social context and social theory in British drugs–crime research. *British Journal of Criminology* 46: 680–703.

Seides R (2010) Should the current DSMIV-TR definition for PTSD be expanded to include serial and multiple micro-traumas as aetiologies. *Journal of Psychiatric and Mental Health Nursing* 17: 725–731.

Select Committee on Science and Technology (1998) *Recreational Use of Cannabis. 9th Report of Select Committee on Science and Technology.* London: House of Lords Publications, ch. 6.

Selten JP, Cantor-Graae E (2005) Social defeat: risk factor for schizophrenia. *British Journal of Psychiatry* 187: 101–102.

Selten JP, Cantor-Graae E (2007) Hypothesis: social defeat is a risk factor for schizophrenia. *British Journal of Psychiatry* 191: 9–12.

Sharfstein SS (2005) Big Pharma and American psychiatry: the good, the bad and the ugly. *Psychiatric News* 40: 3.

Shepherd M (1996) Sir Aubrey Lewis, 1900–1975. *American Journal of Psychiatry* 153: 1624.

Shevlin M, Dorahy MJ, Adamson G (2007a) Trauma and psychosis: an analysis of the National Co-morbidity Survey. *American Journal of Psychiatry* 164: 166–169.

Shevlin M, Dorahy MJ, Adamson G (2007b) Childhood traumas and hallucinations: an analysis of the National Co-Morbidity Survey. *Journal of Psychiatric Research* 41: 222–228.

Smith DJ, Griffiths E, Kelly M, *et al.* (2011) Unrecognised bipolar disorder in primary care patients with depression. *British Journal of Psychiatry* 199: 49–56.

Snowdon CJ (2010) *The Spirit Level Delusion.* London: Little Dice/Democracy Institute.

South London and Maudsley NHS Foundation Trust and South West and St George's Mental Health NHS Trust (2010) *Recovery is for All. Hope, Agency and Opportunity in Psychiatry. A Position Statement by Consultant Psychiatrists.* London: SLAM/SWLSTG.

St John PD, Snow WM, Tyas SL (2010) Alcohol use among older adults. *Reviews in Clinical Gerontology* 20: 56–68.

Stevens A (2007) When two dark figures collide: evidence and discourse on drug related crime. *Critical Social Policy* 27: 77–99.

Stevens A (2008) Weighing up crime: the over estimation of drug related crime. *Contemporary Drug Problems* 35: 265–290.

Stowkowy J, Addington J (2012) Maladaptive schemas as a mediator between social defeat and positive symptoms in young people at clinical high risk for psychosis. *Early Intervention in Psychiatry* 6: 87–90.

Summerfield D (1999) A critique of seven assumptions behind psychological trauma programmes in war-affected areas. *Social Science and Medicine* 48: 1449–1462.

Summerfield D (2000) Childhood, war, refugeedom and 'trauma': three core questions for mental health professionals. *Transcultural Psychiatry* 37: 417–433.

Summerfield D (2001) The invention of post-traumatic stress disorder and the social usefulness of a psychiatric category. *British Medical Journal* 322: 95–98.

Summerfield D (2008) How scientifically valid is the knowledge base of global mental health? *British Medical Journal* 336: 992–994.

Sundquist K, Gölin F, Sundquist J (2004) Urbanisation and incidence of psychosis and depression. *British Journal of Psychiatry* 184: 293–298.

Szasz T (1966) The insanity plea and the insanity verdict. *Temple Law Quarterly* 40: 271.

Szasz T (2007) *The Medicalisation of Everyday Life: Selected Essay.* New York: Syracuse University Press.

Szreter S (1984) The genesis of the Registrar-General's social classification of occupations. *British Journal of Sociology* 35: 522–546.

Torrey EF, Bartko JJ, Lun Z-R, Yolken RH (2007) Antibodies to *Toxoplasma Gondii* in patients with schizophrenia: a meta-analysis. *Schizophrenia Bulletin* 33: 729–736.

Torrey EF, Bowler A (1990) Geographical distribution of insanity in America: evidence for an urban factor. *Schizophrenia Bulletin* 16: 591–604.

Trauer T, Farhall J, Newton R, Cheung P (2001) From long stay psychiatric hospital to community care unit: evaluation at one year. *Social Psychiatry and Psychiatric Epidemiology* 36: 416–419.

Tsuang MT, Stone WS, Faraone SV (2001) Genes, environment and schizophrenia. *British Journal of Psychiatry* 178: 18–24.

Tudor Hart J (1971) The Inverse Care Law. *Lancet* 297: 405–412.

Turner-Crowson J, Wallcraft J (2002) The recovery vision for mental health services and research: a British perspective. *Psychiatric Rehabilitation Journal* 25: 245–254.

Van Os J (2004) Does the urban environment cause psychosis? *British Journal of Psychiatry* 184: 287–288.

Van Os J, Bak M, Hanssen M, *et al.* (2002) Cannabis use and psychosis: a longitudinal population-based study. *American Journal of Epidemiology* 156: 319–327.

Varese F, Smeets F, Drukker M, *et al.* (2012) Childhood adversities increase the risk of psychosis: a meta-analysis of patient–control, prospective and cross-sectional cohort studies. *Schizophrenia Bulletin* 38: 661–671.

Walsh E, Buchanan A, Fahy T (2002) Violence and schizophrenia: examining the evidence. *British Journal of Psychiatry* 180: 490–495.

Walthery P (2006) Figuring out social classes: an overview. *Radical Statistics* 92: 23–40.

Warburton H, Turnbull PJ, Hough M (2005) *Occasional and Controlled Heroin Use: Not a Problem?* York: Joseph Rowntree Foundation.

Warner M, Chen LH, Makuc DM, Anderson RN, Miniño AM (2011) Drug poisoning deaths in the United States, 1980–2008. *NCHS Data Brief* 81: 1–8.

Watts G (2012) Thomas Stephen Szasz. *Lancet* 380: 1380.

Webber M, Huxley P, Harris T (2011) Social capital and the course of depression: six month prospective cohort study. *Journal of Affective Disorders* 129: 149–157.

Welham J, Isohanni M, Jones P, McGrath J (2009) The antecedents of schizophrenia: a review of birth cohort studies. *Schizophrenia Bulletin* 35: 603–623.

Wessely S, Powell R (1989) Fatigue syndromes: a comparison of chronic 'post-viral' fatigue with neuro-muscular and affective disorders. *Journal of Neurology, Neurosurgery and Psychiatry* 52: 940–948.

Wilkinson R, Pickett K (2009) *The Spirit Level: Why More Equal Societies Almost Always Do Better.* London: Allen Lane.

Wilson EO (1975) *Sociobiology: The New Synthesis.* Cambridge, MA: Harvard University Press.

World Heath Organization (2004) *WHO Global Status Report on Alcohol 2004.* Geneva: WHO.

Yolken RH, Dickerson FB, Torrey EF (2009) Toxoplasma and schizophrenia. *Parasite Immunology* 31: 706–771.

Yur'yev A, Värnik A, Värnik P, Sisask M, Leppik L (2012) Employment status influences suicide mortality in Europe. *International Journal of Social Psychiatry* 58: 62–68.

Zammit S, Allebeck P, Andreasson S, Lewis G (2002) Self reported cannabis use as a risk factor for schizophrenia in Swedish conscripts of 1969: historical cohort study. *British Medical Journal* 325: 1199–1201.

Zammit S, Lewis G, Rasbash J, *et al.* (2010) Individuals, schools and neighbourhood: a multilevel longitudinal study of variation in incidence of psychotic disorders. *Archives of General Psychiatry* 67: 914–922.

Zammit S, Spurlock G, Williams H, *et al.* (2007) Genotype effects of *CHRNA7*, *CNR1* and *COMT* in schizophrenia: interactions with tobacco and cannabis use. *British Journal of Psychiatry* 191: 402–407.

Index

Note: page numbers in **bold** refer to boxes, those with suffix 'n' refer to footnotes.